Believe
The Holy Grail of Weight Loss

Your Beliefs
Your Truths
Your Signs
Your God

Your Way Is The Only Way.

Published by World Audience, Inc.
(www.worldaudience.org)
303 Park Avenue South, Suite 1440
New York, NY 10010-3657
Phone (646) 620-7406; Fax (646) 620-7406
info@worldaudience.org
ISBN 978-1-935444-14-5
©2011, Armando Aversa

Copyright notice: All work contained within is the sole copyright of its author, 2011, and may not be reproduced without consent. World Audience (www.worldaudience.org) is a global consortium of artists and writers, producing quality books and the literary journal *Audience*. Please submit your stories, poems, paintings, photography, or artwork: submissions@worldaudience.org. Thank you.

Scripture verses are quoted from *The Holy Bible, New International Version*, copyright 1973, 1978, 1984, by International Bible Society, used by permission of Zondervan; and www.openbible.com.

Believe
Dedicated to mothers,
Discovered for humankind.

Believe **is not about me. This true story I share with you was meant for you to experience. *Believe* is about you and your success.** *Believe* is not a religious movement. I respect you and your religious beliefs, no matter how different from what is expressed in this book. If you are Christian, the true story you are about to read contains many familiar ideas. If you are of a different faith, there are many truths in this message that could apply to all people. At the center of Christian faith is a shared, universal truth that is powerful. In this shared universal truth is the answer.

Do you *Believe* every day is a new beginning, every moment can be a new awakening, and any moment can be a turning point in your life? Your choices, your thoughts, your journey are unique, and you are one of a kind. If you have lost your way but *Believe* a greater purpose influences and drives your life, you are blessed. Truth is, we all have a greater purpose to our lives. The choice is ours to search for and acknowledge our purpose. You are not a victim of circumstances beyond your control; any aspect of your life can be changed by changing the cause that created it, and that cause is located in your mind. Inside your mind and heart is a door no human can shut waiting for you to fully open. Therefore, by mastering your mind, you can attain mastery over any circumstance.

How does one reach his or her divine destiny? There is an answer, an answer that comes with a weight loss approach that leads directly to your success. You are about to discover how your way is the only way!

My journey took ten years; in a moment, you will gain access to my journey and discoveries, the ultimate truths to overcoming any and every struggle you may have with weight loss.

Imagine searching for the ultimate answer to weight loss, an approach every person who believes can accomplish—any weight loss, 100% of the time—and during your quest for this ultimate answer, you see the following image in the sky.

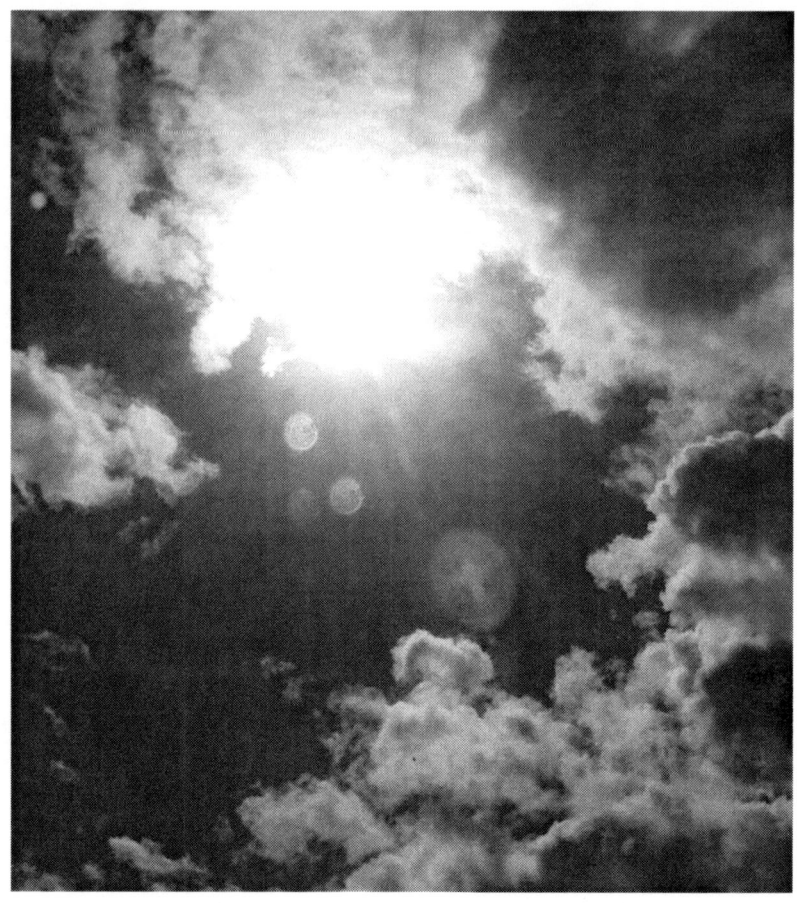

    This is an actual photo taken during the journey to discover the Holy Grail of weight loss. I undertook the journey for you, for each of you who are in search of the truth and your divine purpose. Once you sip from the Holy Grail, your weight loss struggles will be answered and become non-existent.

    I share with you the journey that not only led me to this sign but to others that are astonishing in their clarity.

    This sign in particular is meant for you who are reading *Believe*. Only you can *Believe*.

    "He who believes and hasn't seen is blessed," said Jesus. John 20:29 NIV

I welcome you to a true story of the discovery of the Holy Grail of weight loss.

Believe offers a truth nestled in reality. The book holds your missing link to losing weight, keeping it off effortlessly, and fulfilling your life's aspirations.

Millions of you reading *Believe* have deep faith. Many of you who *Believe* are also struggling with weight loss—not because you lack faith but because you have been misinformed; you haven't yet heard the ultimate solution to your struggles. What if you could use your deepest belief to guide you in reaching your weight loss goals? No matter what state of mind you are currently in—driven by faith or quietly searching—you have the ability to free yourself in a waking moment. Do you *Believe* in signs from above? If you *Believe*, you picked up this book for a reason far greater than just because, you have tapped into your inner spirit.

I, Armando Aversa, promise you that what you are about to read is true, not made up or enhanced in anyway. We now have a connection—you picked up a book I wrote for you, and our connection is not random or accidental: you have in your hands the first sign of a string of signs that will point, ultimately, to your weight loss and your improved health and happiness.

Whether you are a man or a woman, regardless of your race, ethnicity, or religious beliefs, I *Believe* we are all created equal, and everyone can learn priceless wisdom from one another. Without learning from those I have crossed paths with and those who are in my life regularly, *Believe* would not have come to life. *Believe* is for each and every one who is willing to hear the truth and apply the truth.

I now give you an affirmation, a mantra, that when diligently applied can help you rise above all temptations. When used by enough people, the message will manifest throughout the world with blinding speed.

"The truth shall set you free." John 8:23 NIV

The transformation begins with hearing the truth and applying the truth. If you have doubts about giving this book a chance, but something in your gut is telling you to keep reading *Believe*, trust your instinct. What you read will change your life at its core—not because of me but because of you hearing and embracing the truth. During your reading or soon after, you will tap into the rejuvenating power of faith—in yourself and of your belief.

Do you trust your instinct and give *this message* a chance or do you walk away?

If you decide to walk away, may your journey take you elsewhere to hear the truth and to find the power and happiness of *Believe*.

If you have chosen to continue…**your answers lie within!**

Introduction

You are a gift to this world, and you hold within you the power to change yourself and this world for the better, to become the light for your family, your friends, and all who are blessed to come across you. Live the life you were meant to live. Be who you were meant to be. Most importantly, be you. **When you change for the better, it isn't change. It's merely you being who you were meant to be.** Seek the truth!

Believe offers wisdom about weight loss and life. If you *Believe* and internalize the truth, all overwhelming feelings of anxiety, stress, deprivation, and angst that keep you chained to your weight will disappear. Imagine living a life free of anxiety, a life filled with peace and joy. It is possible, and the choice is entirely yours. *You* will conquer any weight loss goal 100% of the time and, as a consequence, thanks to mothers and all who are blessed with hearing the truth, we will help conquer our country's and the world's adult and childhood obesity epidemic.

Think about this: the amount of pounds people have gained, or lost and then regained, most likely far surpasses the total population of America.

Why haven't weight loss programs, systems, or diets worked for you or our country? Perhaps they have worked—for a short time—but then it is extremely difficult to keep the weight off after one loses it. Many diets work, but why has there not been one that works for everyone? Is there one solution to overcoming weight gain or achieving weight loss that lasts a lifetime?

Absolutely!

You could be like most everyone else and follow a diet, system, or program your entire life and hope for success. Once you get the great results you are looking for, then you will most likely fight for the rest of your life to keep the weight off. Your weight loss will be "weight pain"—a constant struggle to maintain the program or system and keep from regaining the pounds. Perhaps this is not the most effective solution. Hence why over 95% of diets have failed the consumer.

Is it possible to lose weight and never feel deprived? To rarely struggle getting rid of the weight and keeping it off. Is it possible to actually enjoy the process?

Yes!

The other solution is not a program or a diet or a system—it's your way of seeing and living the truth, of gaining wisdom and being receptive, of changing your negative habits to positive ones. The other solution won't fail. The other solution won't require you to sacrifice and be uncomfortable. The other solution is the only true solution!

One form of insanity, by definition, is repeating the same actions and expecting a different result—but always getting the same result.

Are we all crazy? Is everyone in our country who is trying to lose weight, participating in crazy fad diets, putting their hard-earned money in the pockets of "professionals," sweating profusely while starving themselves crazy?

Yes. But we are not all insane. We just haven't found the truth, a truth that will reverse habits and choices that have lead to weight gain and a less fulfilling life. Out of the thousands, not a single program, system, diet, fad, or gimmick has conquered our adult and childhood obesity epidemic. Not one solution has reversed the upward trend of our country gaining weight. Obesity is one of the largest epidemics in the entire world. Approximately 70% of adults in the United States are obese or overweight; approximately 30% of our precious children are also obese or overweight as a result of poor modeling by adults. According to studies, 300 million people worldwide are considered obese, and close to 1 billion are overweight. The global number of kids five and younger who are obese is as high as 22 million, and you can imagine the amount of children who are overweight.

We adults need to take control of this epidemic and lead by example. We don't need to get on a diet or follow a program. We can lead by example. Our children look up to us, and it's time to lead them in the right direction. Actions speak louder than words, and our actions are the cure for childhood obesity.

High fat foods, sugary sodas, sedentary lifestyles, high calorie snacks, and hidden calories all contribute to weight gain. As a culture, we have allowed ourselves to wallow in indulgences. When we can't have our sweets and processed foods regularly, we tend to feel deprived. Deprived! Are we serious? We feel deprived when we can't eat sweets daily or when food isn't heaped on our plate for each meal, but we are, in fact, depriving ourselves of eating what our bodies were meant to eat and living a healthy and fulfilled life.

We can reverse the trend toward obesity. Women and those who are mothers who hear and act on the truth and take a stand against the lies and misleading marketing that encourages us to overindulge, to eat too much and too much of the wrong kinds of food, can reverse this epidemic. We can seek the truth and embrace a new, fresh way of seeing ourselves. Of course, mothers want to be healthy for themselves, but they have an additional motivating factor for getting healthy: a love that is strong and so real for their children.

Now all our country needs is a solution that always works. Imagine a single approach that will guide individuals toward a solution guaranteed to work. *Believe* is that imagined solution made real.

Unfortunately, millions in our society are stressed, saddened, depressed, pessimistic, and short-sighted. Over time, our society has stagnated spiritually due to living by false beliefs, beliefs that false prophets like television and movies have given us. Our collective depression and spiritual emptiness are one of the main reasons our country is in a recession and what has caused our society the inability to shed pounds: our social disruption, our unhappiness, and our withering faith are inextricably tied to our weight gain and are leading us down a path where we are destined to struggle and fail.

I have often heard, "people aren't perfect" and "we should be okay with our imperfection." Does that mean we should not try to change the flaws that are limiting us? We are all born pure, but time and society can corrupt us if we allow it to. Each individual can change course and can navigate away from these impurities of mind and character. Naturally, we make poor decisions, but the poorest decision is being unwilling to alter one's course and choices. Some of us give up on ourselves, believing we can never change and that life has dealt us bad cards. Perhaps we make the excuse that our unhappiness, our extra weight, is not our fault—and we blame others. In some ways, it is not our fault—we have not yet heard the truth and have fallen into a way of thinking that is destructive. We are all vulnerable to the pessimism that infects our world; we are all vulnerable to advertisers who trick us into believing we need, we must have, we are desperate for this or that unhealthy food or behavior. But we are all also strong enough to resist and form new ways of thinking and feeling.

Fortunately, you and millions of others have deep faith and haven't given up. Fortunately, there are those who will grasp the truth of this message and become empowered. Fortunately, there are those who *Believe*! We believers have the opportunity to turn that unfortunate tide. We can conquer obesity, and you will lose weight and keep it off!

So what is the answer to your weight loss success?

The renewal of your mind.

The power of our mind is amazing. By simply creating new thought processes, one can transform and replace misguided beliefs. At any moment, a revelation can strike. A developed conscious awareness will turn into a heightened awareness that leaves one feeling accomplished before even starting the journey. The empowered feeling is the beauty of believing in your approach, in yourself, and in your God. Our minds hold the key to conquering, to vanquishing our struggles with weight loss and life. New ways of thinking will propel us into our lives, enriching every aspect of our world.

***Believe* is not about me. This true story I share with you was meant for you to experience. *Believe* is about you and your success.** The wisdom in *Believe's* message will revolutionize every aspect of your life; yes, you will lose and keep weight off, but all aspects of your life will flourish.

The truths of *Believe* are in the story, the story of a journey toward the ultimate truth to weight loss. I could offer you a diet plan like many other programs offer, provide you a specific protocol for when and what to eat; I could tell you the secret of weight loss right now in a simple, bumper-sticker aphorism. But neither would work.

To enjoy a spiritually rich and meaningful, healthy life, your beliefs have to become a reality; you will tap in to your power when you internalize your beliefs and make them the foundation for your way of life. Our beliefs, when they are of the truth, will be the scaffolding for the beautiful structure of our lives; if we continue to harbor beliefs that are pessimistic the negative power will hinder one's ability to reach weight loss goals and life's aspirations.

I dedicate *Believe* to mothers, but the power of this discovery is for all who choose to embrace it.

Believe: is for anyone who is seeking a more satisfying, empowered life. For those who are seeking the life we were meant to live: a message of comfort, goodness, and purity. A weight loss theory for everyone that enriches all aspects of life. An approach that will never fail you.

This is a true story that will plug you into the electric current of faith, wisdom, and the power of believing.

Believe is one of the most powerful words ever created. Belief in seeking the truth, in gaining knowledge and wisdom, is what will allow the truth to set you free. Belief in negative thinking will cripple one's soul. Imagine reaching your weight loss goal and enjoying the journey along the way. Imagine discovering your divine destiny. Imagine living in utter peace daily!

Let's walk together toward wisdom and insight through a journey of the subconscious.

My heart is with each and every one of you who apply principles of truth to your life and live the life you were meant to live.

Anything is possible when you *Believe* ...

> *"Then you will know truth*
> *and the truth shall set you free."* John 8:32 NIV

Sit back, relax, and enjoy the journey. *Believe...*

1.
Patience

I have been inspired by others my entire life and am grateful to have come across people of all backgrounds. These experiences are what have made *Believe* possible.

Before you continue to read, please find a quiet place, a place you will want to remember. Take your time to embrace and ponder the story. Put yourself in my shoes, **live the moments** with me, and **consider what you would do**. Walk the journey with me and discover the missing links to your success and the renewal of your mind.

Believe is not about me; it's about you, and the journey I embarked on was for you to hear and see. I feel fortunate to have the opportunity through this story for you to get to know who I am and how my feelings and thoughts arose. It is you who are blessed because you are willing to hear and embrace the truth.

I received a phone call on December 8, 2009, from a close friend who invited me to visit Dallas, Texas. I was reluctant to go, but something inside told me to take the trip. Work, family, the list of to do's, the lack of money, and everything going on in my life at the time said not to go, but how can I deny my gut instinct?

Luckily, I did go. If I hadn't taken the trip, the journey you are about to read would likely never have happened and *Believe* wouldn't have been born.

While packing my things for Dallas, I included a letter I had saved from a client. I did not open the letter when I first received it a few weeks prior. Luckily, I've evolved into a very patient person; I was waiting for the right moment. I don't tend to save letters, but I do trust my instincts; when my gut tells me to do or not to do something, I listen. Something told me not to open the letter the day Debbie gave it to me, to wait until the time was right. I patiently waited. I brought the unopened letter with me on my journey to Texas.

I arrived in Dallas in the late afternoon. Waiting for me at the airport was my close friend Jon, his wife Tina, and his business partner, Jacob. We embraced with warm hugs, and from that moment, I instantly had a feeling the trip was going to be special and unforgettable. I experienced a strong sense of destiny! Jacob and I had only met once previously, and we had an instant connection. We shared a passion about the health and well-being of others, a passion similar to a mother's passion toward her own children. Such a strong sentiment in two men may sound hard to *Believe*, but we shared a strong bond—we both understood and appreciated the kindness and wisdom mothers bring to the world.

Jon and Jacob established a company that is currently among the elite in the health industry. I have known Jon since the beginning of high school; even then, he had a belief, a belief to follow his passion. He never gave up on what he believed; despite hardship and doubters, he remained true to his convictions, and his dream became reality. Jon had the kind of passion that fills one's soul by simply believing! Watching him succeed led me to a deeper belief in the possibilities of how we can overcome our obstacles or setbacks. Jon strived to learn and grow, and his patience and desire defeated any temporary negative feelings.

When I arrived in Dallas, I saw Jon and Jacob's incredible success. Jon's success shouldn't have been much of a surprise, but I was in shock. In a matter of a brief time, he surged from his role as a personal trainer to establishing one of the leading companies in the health industry. Imagine that! His rise is a feat that will remain in history as one of the fastest growing and most reputable companies ever created in the industry.

They were two people who lived on opposite ends of the country and were united by coming across one another on a blog. They both shared a passion, desire, and a dream to help millions of people improve their lives not by lying or misleading but by creating amazing products. Jon and Jacob are living out their passions by helping others achieve theirs. Priceless!

Life is all about finding your passions. Isn't it? Or is it about living a robotic life where society's messages will eventually lead us astray? We can easily lose ourselves in society's negative messages. Unfortunately, life has become an uninspired drudgery for many. Such mindlessness is not entirely our fault; the world's way creates delusions into routines and habits that are destructive—intentionally or not, our daily routines can create false truths that lead us astray. Millions of people, on a day to day basis, are being stripped of hopes and dreams. Unfortunately, we have become a country that has been misinformed and mislead about weight loss and life. Together, from one individual to the next, we can shatter the drudgery our society has created. It is up to individuals to restore their desire. Personal lethargy and weight gain won't disappear because other companies will stop lying and misleading us but because you will be able to spot the truth.

Knowingly or not, we all are passionate about something—you have a spark that you hope the daily routines will not smother. If you know your passion, ultimately it is your choice whether you pursue making your dream a reality or if you allow the dream to slip away. Why not seek the truth behind your purpose in life? We were all put on this planet for a reason, a reason far greater than we may ever know. Fortunately, if one desires to seek, we have a way to find our deeper purpose in life, and that purpose lies within the mindset needed to overcome weight loss.

Sometimes, we bump into someone or have an unexpected discovery that changes the course of our lives, and we can call these coincidences or signs of a larger destiny, a larger plan. Sometimes, we make mistakes or experience failures, and some call these setbacks—or opportunities for growth and expansion. Depending on the language we use to describe life's events, our unique experiences can be positive or negative. Luckily, I chose the positive. Always! Why? You are about to see.

One of my purposes for the visit to Dallas was to show Jacob some training secrets to maximizing muscle contraction during an exercise and how to get better results when working out in the same amount of time. Being a personal trainer for the past ten years, I have developed a keen eye and obsession for optimizing form during an exercise. You might ask, why? Well, if I or a client is going to spend time resistance training, it only makes sense to get 100% out of every exercise being performed. Anything else would not only be a waste of time but would yield fewer results and eventually accrue the possibility of joint pain. Improper and inefficient form is very common amongst those who weight train. Look around the next time you are in a gym at how differently each person performs the same exercise. These are exercises that should be performed only one way, but yet individuals vary greatly in their approach. Think about the time one is wasting, the results one is missing out on, and the possible joint pain one may be accruing. It just doesn't make sense not to make the most of one's time and get the most out of one's workout.

When we first arrived at the gym, I asked Jacob to show me the most common exercises he performs on a regular basis. He proceeded to show me a variety of common exercises. For the most part, like millions of others, ten out of the ten exercises he performed could be enhanced in a way to encourage more muscle recruitment (better results)! I would say nearly 100% of people weight training can enhance their form and achieve better results. The math is simple: if you perform an exercise only 80 or 90% correctly, you are missing out on 10-20% of every rep, every set, everyday you are in a gym. It's amazing when you think about how much time one wastes in the gym—and the lack of great results one could be achieving!

When I showed Jacob a few key elements to change, he felt an immediate, dramatic difference. He was blown away! Now, we're talking about somebody who exercises regularly and who was intrigued by the instant feeling he got from making small adjustments. He couldn't *Believe* the difference he felt and said, "Armando, there are millions who workout and need this information. I have never seen or heard of these little details. I'm in shock."

I was ecstatic and thought in my head, did he just say millions?

Jacob said, "Would you create a DVD? We will link it to our product line." I thought about it for a half a second and said, "Of course! I'd be honored."

Imagine that! I was asked to create a DVD to help millions better utilize their time and enhance their results. I have always been passionate about helping others, and now I had the opportunity to reach millions! I knew the DVD would be an instant success. I would have the unique opportunity to share information about proper form that few in the world had ever seen. Unfortunately, working out and doing cardio is not the main solution to weight loss. One would have to work out for hours every day to overcome poor eating habits. Of course, I'm delighted to help others learn how to work out more efficiently, but exercise is only one small part of the ultimate solution.

I felt like my trip was already a success, but little did I know what was about to happen next.

We went out that night to celebrate the purchase of Jon and Jacob's new homes. I couldn't get it out of my mind that the CEO of a company at the top of its industry was impressed with the tips I had offered him. I was ecstatic that one of my passions in life was going to be fulfilled.

The next morning when I woke, everyone was still sleeping. Apparently, we had enjoyed the evening since it was close to noon. I was sitting in a recliner in the middle of a room overlooking the skyline of downtown Dallas, an amazing view. As I enjoyed the scenery, I watched the sun creep between two skyscrapers. The sun fit perfectly within the two skyscrapers as if the buildings were perfectly placed or God had perfectly placed the sun. I lay my head back on the chair with my eyes closed and felt the warmth of the sun on my face. It was a record low of 17 degrees outside, but it felt as if I were in the Caribbean. The feeling and warmth of the sun was breathtaking.

I enjoyed this moment thoroughly while I was thinking of the future. Quite suddenly, I felt a strong heat overtake my body.

I had never experienced such calm, potent warmth. The energy was unquestionably real. I simply could not ignore the sun's touch. I felt as if God were sending me a message. Without thinking, I reached into my briefcase and pulled out the letter my client Debbie had given me. As I mentioned, I saved her words for when the time felt right, and with what felt to be God's warmth surging through my body, I felt no time could be better.

I looked at the scenery and the sun one more time.

I took a deep breath and opened the letter:

Dear Armando,

I recently asked myself, "how is it that you, Armando, were able to help me conquer my greatest hurdle in life when nothing up until this point helped me to do that?" I have used food and alcohol as a crutch for most of my life. Some stages were worse than others, but I ate and drank as a way to deal with my stress. Along with my struggle with alcohol and poor food choices, I continued to struggle with my relationship with God. For some reason, those two things were completely related.

As an adult, I chose to stay home when my children were born. In a society that values job titles and salaries, this had a great impact on my self-esteem and feelings of self worth. And I continued to drink and overeat to mitigate those negative feelings. I spent countless hours and thousands of dollars on self-help books, diet books, trainers, and therapists, trying to "fix" myself. Then, somewhere along the line in the hours of speaking with you, I found the courage to stop using alcohol and food as a coping mechanism. As a result of that, I now feel God's presence so completely and so powerfully, it has been life changing.

As a college educated Exercise Science major, your technical knowledge of resistance training is superior. Certainly seeing physical results gave me some initial confidence, but it was more than that. In the business of helping people, you understand human nature. But you did not gain your insight through text books, Master's degrees, and PhD's but rather by working tens of thousands of hours in the trenches along with the women you have come across. You have dedicated your life to learning about women, understanding their struggles, feeling their pain, listening to them talk longingly about missed opportunities and unrealized dreams. You have embraced every story, every broken heart and lost soul, internalized it, and emerged as the man you are today. The one man capable of helping me unlock my true potential and the potential of millions of women in search of the truth. Gone is the weak, insecure woman who was "just a mom." Now when I look in the mirror, I see a strong, confident woman with value and purpose. Thanks to you, I now view my role as a mother as more important than the most prestigious CEO positions.

When I met you, my first thought was, "How does a personal trainer afford a million dollar home and a full-sized gym in his house?" Fully embracing my own negativity and skepticism, I immediately suspected that you must come from money and have led a charmed life. I was surprised to learn that I couldn't have been more wrong! When I learned the process you took of building your house without any experience, I was simply in shock! You were not born with a silver spoon in your mouth, but instead you were instilled with an incredible work ethic, someone for whom there is no such word as can't, and a person with a true optimistic outlook on life in every and all situations. Your lifestyle, your energy, and your passion were things I wanted for myself but thought it would always be out of reach for me. Clearly, I was wrong and soon found it was possible and easier than I ever dreamed.

Armando, becoming a trainer was not a career choice for you, but a divinely inspired calling. For me, the greatest benefit through all of this has been my renewed relationship with God and my family. Because your life, words, and wisdom have had such a transformational effect on me, my husband and children have responded to my new positive outlook in similar fashion. They view the world with new excitement and passion, in search of reaching their goals and fulfilling their dreams. WHAT MORE COULD ANY MOTHER ASK FOR? :) Your spirit, your soul, and your words are simply beautiful and one of a kind. Imagine the impact on our society if every mother had the opportunity to hear your message. Armando, like you said time and time again, it is through mothers that this world will conquer our nations adult and child obesity epidemic!

God has clearly chosen you to work this miracle in my life and the life of others. I have new goals and new dreams, and I am accomplishing all of them! None of this would have been possible without you. There is something about your spirit and soul…something that reaches people on a different level. I know you will reach a level of success that most people only dream about. When they hear your words, then their dreams can and most definitely will become a reality. God is using you, Armando to reach all the women in the world who are in search of the guidance to reclaiming their lives. They deserve nothing less than the opportunity to hear your words and receive your gift.

Sincerely,
Debbie Bohling

P.S. There are many amazing things happening in my life right now. There's no doubt in my mind, Armando, that you are connected to all of it. You have a special gift that the world needs. It is now your time to release your words to those women in this world in search of who they were meant to be!

After reading Debbie's letter, my emotions took hold of me, and my body began to tremble. My eyes filled with tears of joy for Debbie and for the millions of mothers in search of the truth. Her letter opened my eyes: what I have been searching for is within. Debbie's words awakened me to the truth of the gift I have within. The moment had never fully crystallized for me prior to reading her words. It was in this moment I believed!

A letter of thanks inspired me to write a book and to reach out to tens of millions. It actually felt as if the book was written and tens of millions were successful. That's the power of believing! I understood at that moment that a small act can incite great change. The world can change for the better if we grasp on to each others' passion, desire and truths. From one person to the next, you just never know how a simple gesture can change one's life.

And from that one life, the change will spread to one another and millions.

Once I got myself together, I texted Debbie to show my appreciation. I couldn't text quickly enough to express my gratitude and to share with her the power of the revelation she had inspired in me:

> Wow! Talk about perfect timing! I am sitting here in Dallas, Texas, with tears rolling down my face, embracing this indescribable feeling. I am blown away with your generous and kind words….simply beautiful! I truly want to thank you from the bottom of my heart for this letter. Reading your words at this time will be a moment I will never forget and one I will cherish forever!
>
> You should be very proud of yourself for what you have accomplished. Many people in this world hide from their truths and feel they can't change or don't want to change for the better. You embraced your truths and believed in yourself. Fortunately, you didn't give up during the process by following a diet. Instead, you persevered and were honest with yourself. You created your own way, and your results will last you a lifetime! You deserve all the credit! You are a beautiful person inside and out and deserve a life filled with indescribable, positive feelings and great fortune. God bless you and your family. I am grateful to have come across such beautiful people.
>
> Thanks to your success and reaching out to me, your letter inspired me to write a book that I am going to dedicate to mothers. A book that

will undoubtedly reach millions and conquer our adult and childhood obesity epidemic.

Imagine that! Within a moment and with absolute conviction, I knew that within the depths of my soul, I held the missing link to the success of hundreds of millions who struggle with weight loss and life.

I decided to put the DVD on hold, to forego all the money and all the material success. I knew I would write a best seller before I even began to put my words on paper.

Although I had one very large obstacle in the way: how in the world could someone who is not an author, someone who doesn't write, and someone who has resisted reading my entire life going to write a book?

Actually, it's simple! I trusted an approach and a way of thinking that will never fail. So where do I start? **The foundation**.

The foundation is the single most important aspect of any undertaking: structurally, physically, and mentally. Without a solid foundation, our dreams will remain inert, un-fulfilled and un-realized. Building the proper foundation in weight loss is the missing link to losing weight and easily keeping it off, forever. Yes, easily! I promise!

What is the foundation? In all honesty, at this moment, I myself didn't even know exactly. *"Seek and you shall find" Matthew 7:7 NIV,* came to mind.

After sending Debbie the text message, I sat back in the chair and reminisced about how a sudden, life-changing decision came about so quickly. I have spent many years investigating the causes of weight gain in hopes of discovering an ultimate truth and answer. I spoke to people from all walks of life. For over thirty thousand hours, I listened to others' stories, learning, assessing, and analyzing. I opened myself to the successes and failures of others' stories of weight gain, weight loss, and struggles in life. Hearing the stories, embracing the smaller truths contained in each individual's struggle and success is what made my dream become attainable.

I believed there was a way to lose weight that wasn't about following a diet but more about finding a larger truth that would allow individuals to reach their divine destiny in life.

I did not decide to go on this journey to seek personal fame and fortune. I decided to seek the truth because I *Believe* everyone should have an opportunity to live an exuberant, meaningful, free life with a deeper purpose and with greater meaning. We can realize our gifts and talents; we shouldn't let them lay dormant within our soul. As adults, it is up to us to create a positive, enriching environment for ourselves, and for our children to grow up in and enjoy a healthy and fulfilled life.

~ Your Personal Notes ~

2.

The seeds of this timeless weight loss theory were planted during the years I played baseball in college. I had a lot of heart as a player; I was enthusiastic and engaged. I wanted to be a professional baseball player and had prospects of moving on past college. I invested every single ounce of energy into making my dream become a reality. The day my dream of playing professional baseball ended, I felt voided. All my energy drained. I became a shell, and I seriously considered ending my life. The ability to realize my dream of becoming a major league baseball player was out of my control: no matter how hard I worked to throw harder, I just couldn't. During the last game of my senior year, I stood in the bullpen and knew my career was over.

I felt the pain and confusion often associated with losing a loved one. The pain, the anger, the thoughts of "why me" were racing through my head. Part of me died. I almost had to be carried off the field. I became depressed, yet no one knew the magnitude of my depression. I couldn't understand why God would take something from me that I was so passionate about. Such irrational cruelty didn't make sense. I dedicated myself to baseball; I poured my soul into improving, and yet God had not granted me the gift to live my dream.

From my earliest memories, baseball provided the core of my sense of self-worth. I assumed I had been created primarily for the purpose of becoming a professional. And yet, suddenly, my dream was over. I wanted to give up. I wanted it all to end.

I am sure many of you who are reading my story have a similar tale to tell and can relate to the emotional devastation I experienced. At some point in your life, have you felt as if you've been stripped of your dreams or goals? Or perhaps you have just lost yourself along the way? Unfortunately, millions feel cheated and despairing.

As I contemplated suicide, I was fortunate to have a moment of revelation. Perhaps I had a different purpose, a greater purpose. Perhaps God had not denied me my destiny but had instead steered me toward a different path. Perhaps my desire to become a professional baseball player was a false desire.

Remarkably, I began to look at the loss of my baseball dreams as an opportunity, an opening to allow a new success to manifest. It didn't make sense to look at the loss of my false dream as a failure; I had been directed to a new path.

For each of us, what looks like failure is truly opportunity. One goal may fail, but another opportunity—a greater, truer opportunity—awaits. If I hadn't suffered the dark night of my soul, if I hadn't played baseball for years with passion and determination, I would not have developed the skills necessary to succeed with my greater mission. Once I knew the truth of my destiny, once I had seen the light of truth and the real path of my life, I was able to redirect my work ethic, dedication, and passion for baseball toward my new life and toward finding the ultimate cure of weight loss.

All along, I thought I had been practicing hitting and pitching, but really I had been practicing skills I could now transfer to solving one of the world's major epidemics with conviction, desire and focus.

I felt freed of a burden. I could see clearly the great qualities I had developed while simultaneously acknowledging all the qualities I didn't posses and weaknesses I held within. Living with such clarity made sense. I made a decision to strive for perfection in all aspects of my life, to grow and evolve in every aspect of my being, knowing I will never be perfect but realizing the real glory comes from the strive toward greatness. Think about this for a minute. I was an impatient person at the time, but why would I want to live life with such anxiety? Over time, I learned being patient is crucial; we can be persistent, but persistently impatient behaviors will not lead to success.

From that moment forward, I learned from my mistakes rather than emphasize self-pity. I now look outside myself, too, and learn from others' mistakes. Why not acknowledge my weaknesses? Why hide from my truths? Why fight against truths? I decided to seek and embrace facts and to live life around the truth. The self-loathing path led to despair and self- annihilation; I was moving toward self-improvement and actualization. Obviously, we all will make mistakes and have setbacks. Mistakes, though, are an opportunity to reveal our character. A key to acquiring power is acknowledging our mistakes and learning from them. Setbacks are successes because we grow from them. I could have given up, allowed myself to wallow in self-pity and negativity—but I would have spent my entire life with those emotions and the consequence of that bad habit. Being negative is a life decision that influences every thought and action we take. I decided I wanted to live in utter peace and that I would seek a better path.

I wasn't meant to be a professional baseball player. And for the first time, acknowledging the truth, I felt okay—and even empowered. Imagine: in one moment, I wanted to kill myself, but in the next I felt revived.

What is my truth? And what are the truths? I didn't know at the time, but I was about to pursue answers: *"Seek the truth as the truth shall set you free." John 8:32 NIV*

~ Your Personal Notes ~

3.

Jacob had just awakened. When he entered the room, our eyes traded a glance. I was still glassy eyed from reading the letter. The look on his face was priceless; he knew something significant had just happened. "Armando, are you ok?"

I said to him, "Bro, you need to read this letter." As he was reading, I could tell Debbie's powerful words touched him. He said, "Wow, Armando. I'm speechless."

He asked how I met Debbie. The crazy thing is, I told him, that I was training her son at first. I asked her one day while she was dropping off her son, if she would be interested in working out with him. She said sure; she would like to give training a try. I asked if she was the same size as she was in college. She told me that in college, she was a size 6, and she at the time was a snug size 12. I said, "If you want to look like you did in college, the transformation will be a lot easier than you might think." She looked at me in disbelief and said, "That would be amazing." She asked, "You're not going to try and change my diet are you? Because there is no way I am going to change the way I eat." I said, "No, don't worry. We'll start to workout and see what happens from there."

"However," I told her, "I'd like you to consider an approach to weight loss that is very different. I guarantee you haven't heard of it, an approach that works 100% of the time with anyone who applies it to his or her life. Regardless of how limited one's time, or how overweight, or how lost one might feel, it's an approach that never fails!"

She smiled, skeptical but willing. She told me she was willing to try something new but confirmed she did not want to change her diet—she liked what and how she ate now. And eating what she does is important to her socially and personally. She claimed to find satisfaction with how she was living her life. I've heard this before a couple of thousand times.

Over the course of our training sessions—boom—she lost over 30lbs of fat, and I received her letter of gratitude and appreciation.

After hearing Debbie's story, Jacob said, "Armando, that's an amazing story. I am dying to hear about your theory!" He sat in a chair across from me. We could both see the sun now creeping toward the top of the buildings.

I shared with him the secret of *Believe*.

"Armando! That is amazing! I have never looked at weight loss in that way. It makes complete sense. I can see why her life changed." He thought for a minute. "I truly *Believe* you have discovered the ultimate answer to weight loss."

"So", I said to Jacob, "Looks like we are going to have to put that DVD on hold. I am on a mission to write a book and dedicate it to mothers that's going to conquer our country's obesity epidemic."

He looked at me and said, "I have no doubt and have all the faith in you and this theory doing just that."

I didn't expect to convince Jacob so easily. He is a man of critical intelligence and keen judgment, but he was as amazed as I. For those who are prepared, seeing and then certifying the truth is easy. He believed! And so did I!

After our conversation, and then as I embarked on my mission to write a book, I felt an amazing peace. I felt as if I accomplished my dream, and yet making my dream real was still far away from happening. My happiness, my peace, was not dependent on achieving the goal but rather on my conviction that my goal was real and that I would make real my desire.

That's the power when one truly believes, when you are certain of the uncertainty, when you just know you know because you know. The majority of those I have trained at first lacked one of the most important elements to one's success in weight loss and life. They lacked a belief that they could lose weight and restore looking and feeling more youthful. They lacked the truth that it is possible to lose weight no matter how old, what size, or how out of shape one is. When we *Believe* in ourselves and the approach we are taking, reaching our goal is inevitable and a certainty. The journey is priceless. Imagine that! Who would think that the journey would be the priceless and enjoyable part? We need to embrace the journey, not dread it. What is learned along the way is far greater than achieving the goal. Why? Because without learning your truths, you will reach your goal without having a clue how to maintain your results.

~ Your Personal Notes ~

4.

When I returned to Connecticut, my life continued with its normal routines and patterns; however, now I felt a serious connection with my inner soul, my motivating self-conscience, a connection so deep and so real I simply could not deny its presence.

I went to bed the first night back at the same time as usual but found myself wide awake at 3am. I cursed my restlessness, knowing I had a group to train at 6am. I attempted to return to sleep, but I couldn't. I lay on my back, awake and thinking, hoping for sleep, until 5:15am and then started my day.

Although the day seemed very different, my mind was renewed, and I was thinking more clearly than ever before.

I felt at peace, and I now knew how utter peacefulness would appear in my daily life. What a joyous, remarkable feeling, a feeling I wish upon everyone. You, too, will have this feeling on the day, the moment you *Believe*. When you *Believe* in yourself, when you *Believe* in what it is you are looking to accomplish and that the path you are taking is the hardened and proven path.

I went to bed, satisfied and peaceful, the next night at the same time as usual and guess what? Yes, I was awake again at 3am. I cussed again, but lightly this time, because I knew my sleeplessness was not generated by anxiety but by excitement and the prospect of success and happiness.

The same pattern recurred for days on end. I was mystified. I had been a sound sleeper all my life, but suddenly I wake at 3am every morning with uncontrollable energy. I began to suspect that my sleeplessness must have a greater significance, that perhaps I was supposed to do something great from 3 – 5 in the morning, that being awake was a gift.

From that realization forward, for the next 3 weeks when I woke in the middle of the night, I spoke and wrote the words that were emerging from the depths of my soul and subconscious. I continued my writing for three weeks, and after three weeks of waking up every morning at 3am, I wasn't the slightest bit tired. I felt I needed a break, but a new source of energy kept me going. I didn't stop writing and talking into a tape recorder.

I didn't want thoughts to come to me by sitting down and forcing them out or thinking about what I needed to say. I was seeking words that came from within. I felt I needed to write this book with the words coming from my subconscious, arriving to me almost as if in a vision; I allowed the thoughts to come to me naturally at any moment, and I listened to the words and recorded them. I knew the thoughts would be more authentic and in turn more genuine; the truth of my approach was streaming out of me, and I had only to bottle the wisdom of my subconscious. Being awake was not a curse. Being awake was an opportunity to listen, to record, and to share the truth of my experience.

I have been a sound sleeper my entire life, enjoying seven to eight hours without fail. Perhaps you are not a sound sleeper; anxiety drives many of us out of bed. We worry, we fuss, and we allow our unhappiness to keep us from visualizing our dreams. Most of the time, our sleeplessness is unproductive, and the resulting lethargy affects our health, our families, and our careers—and keeps us from reaching our divine purpose.

I also became someone who couldn't sleep, but I chose not to pity myself; rather, I saw the extra hours as an opportunity to capture and make real my dream. I felt invigorated. My sleeplessness also affected me, but I chose to not think negatively.

If you are someone who only wishes you could sleep, trust that sound, quality sleep will happen one day, the day you put your mind at peace. I am fortunate. I had an "Oh, my God!" moment and realized the blessing of my wakefulness rather than wallowing in self-pitying and feeling like I had been cheated. I shifted my perspective to see the positive in what could easily been seen as a negative. I turned on a light rather than cursing the darkness. After all, how would I write a book after 10 hours of working? It made sense to me for me to write after some rest.

My writing and recording in the early morning is the core of the core, the **foundation**. I needed to get all my thoughts on paper or on a recorder, capturing every thought at any moment, thoughts of purity and of truth.

Just like in weight loss; the most important aspect is our foundation. The foundation we lay is the most important, most key aspect to accomplishing our weight loss goals. Establish a solid, positive foundation where you shift from negative to positive thoughts, where you see opportunity instead of loss, where you turn yourself from victim into aggressor; plain and simple. Once you establish your foundation, the core principles will color all parts of your life.

Without the core foundational shift in attitude, you will vacillate between weight loss and gain. You will continually fight negative thoughts and self-pity that will keep you from attaining your goals. Imagine losing weight but always feeling deprived, always struggling to keep it off. What's the point, right? Without a foundation, demonstrating intermittent will-power and following a diet or program will never work. We are doomed to fall back into a cycle of regret, believing we are victims. Following a diet, program, or system can be beneficial, but the results are often temporary. To lose weight and keep the pounds off, developing your foundation is the key!

I'm not going to tell you constructing a foundation—so different from what we have been taught to *Believe*, so different from the negative viewpoint our culture tends to embrace—is easy. But I will tell you that no matter who you are, creating a strong foundation is always possible when we fully embrace the truth of your belief. Only you can make the connection and accomplish the transformation. The foundation is a learned behavior that anyone can implement with daily, conscious awareness. Eventually your conscious awareness becomes who you are. You begin thinking without thinking. The reason why millions remain overweight and many succeed only short term or painfully try to keep weight off is because they have failed to construct a solid foundation.

Imagine a solution that works 100% of the time, a solution that never fails! There is one, and it's not just eating healthy and exercising. Are you just dying to know? I would be too, but you see at this point, I still didn't even know the truth myself. I knew I had the answers for assessing individual clients, but I hadn't discovered the words to put on paper before you. I had to continue to seek the truth millions need to know and fully embrace. What Jacob had heard in Dallas that sunny morning was only a skeleton of the idea. I needed the flesh, the muscle. At the time, I only explained part of my theory because I needed to continue to seek.

I might have thought I was done, but no wisdom worth believing, no truth powerful enough to enhance lives of millions is so easily attained. I had more of the path to walk, and so do you with me.

~ Your Personal Notes ~

5.

I continued to work nonstop throughout the day and night, but then I hit a wall. I was exhausted—excited, but worn. I needed to regroup and give my mind a break. I wanted to continue to work, but I also felt inspired to get away. Something within me felt I should go to one of my favorite places Newport, Rhode Island. Newport is stunning. Picture tens of miles of pristine landscape along the Atlantic. Green, lush, beautiful lawns stretch along cliffs that provide a barrier from the ocean's waves. The sights are truly breathtaking.

I have always admired the beauty of landscapes. I have tremendous appreciation and gratitude for what this earth provides us—from the scenery to the people and the beautiful foods grown in her fertile soil. Perhaps we could see the land as bitter or unforgiving or even barren, but simple gratitude leads us toward the positive, toward the lush and generous world that nurtures, protects, and motivates us. When you embrace the truth about the benefits of the foods this earth provides, you become humbled; it's an honor to know how lucky we truly are. Fruits, vegetables, fish, whole grains, and legumes possess cancer fighting agents, disease preventing properties, stress reducing nutrients, and fat burning properties—they are truly remarkable! Healthy foods are essential, and when we embrace the truth of their value and goodness, we move closer to embracing the truth.

Over the years, I have struggled with weight gain at times. Nearly every time, I was focusing on what I wasn't eating instead of having gratitude for the magnificent foods that were available to me. I decided to focus on the positive and acknowledge the truth that eating healthy rather than indulging in less nutritious foods was a necessary part of life.

When you gain knowledge of what the earth offers us, you will develop an appreciation for the richness and bounty of healthy options we have available—truly, we are blessed! If you eat healthy foods and maintain a healthy weight, you can expect to have a lot more energy, stronger immune system, healthier eyes, skin, hair and nails, improved sex drive, sharper mental focus, stronger blood and respiratory systems, decrease the signs of aging. God's bounty provides fiber, vitamins, and antioxidants rich in phytochemicals that help prevent certain diseases such as cancer, heart disease, strokes, high blood pressure, osteoporosis, high cholesterol, diabetes, hormonal imbalance, polycystic ovarian disease, infertility, sleep apnea, chronic inflammation, cellular damage, arterial stiffness and, of course, weight gain.

Alternately, when one eats unhealthy foods, the risks begin to mount: chronic or life-threatening illnesses such as diabetes, coronary heart disease, obstructed arteries, weight gain, obesity, atherosclerosis, hypertension, angina, strokes, heart attack, kidney failure, type 2 diabetes, osteoarthritis, sleep apnea, cancer, thyroid dysfunction, intestinal problems, gum diseases, muscle deterioration, vision loss and depression most likely will develop. The list of negative factors is endless.

When we eat healthy foods, we are nurturing our bodies; when we eat unhealthily, we are depriving our bodies of the nutrients necessary to function optimally and be healthy. Feel deprived because you can't eat sweets daily? Don't! Eating sweets daily deprives you of numerous health benefits and provides you with only serious, long-term negative health consequences.

Newport is full of energy as well as peace and quietness. I was heading toward The Cliff Walk where the roar of the ocean contributes to a sense of peace. I was grateful to have a client and friend offer me her house for the weekend. Before leaving, I decided to ask another friend if she would like to join me. Michelle was a client who had recently lost 35 pounds. When I first met her, she was depressed and saddened by many things that had happened in her life. Fortunately she saw the same beauty within her that I saw when she asked for help. She found a deeper meaning to her life. She wrote me a letter about her transformation:

Dear Armando,

When I first came to you, I was a completely different person. I was someone who was in such a deep hole that all I saw was darkness. I had no self-worth. I was ashamed, hurt, full of hate and anger. I was a lost, overweight person. It's not that I wanted to kill myself. I just felt lifeless. I was beaten by someone who I once loved. I had two knee surgeries while in my twenties that hindered my ability to workout because all it did was aggravate my knee even more. I was always someone who loved life and loved loving others, but that person no longer existed. She was ripped away from me. I'm sure most women could relate to my story. I often overlooked things in the past and didn't want to recognize my new condition, so I buried it deep within and moved forward. I then continued down the same road of misery and a feeling of being uncomfortable in my own skin. I always felt sorry for myself. I put up a wall, always feeling attacked and nothing but angry all the time. I gained a ton of weight and lost the shape of the beautiful, athletic legs I once had. My legs were surrounded by fat, and I was so ashamed and embarrassed of them. This was no way to live life at 29 years old, weighing over 160 pounds and only 5'4". I mean, come on.

When I first came to you, I knew right away there was something about you I trusted. It wasn't because of your good looks or the reputation you had built for yourself of being a personal trainer. I felt something, an energy that I had never felt before when meeting someone for the first time. I trusted you and opened up to you with things that paper has never seen before. When talking to you, you never told me what to do, you never asked me to change, you didn't create me, you didn't mold me--you just spoke and guided me. There was one day that I remember specifically what you said, and that's when the switch went on, "You can be whoever you were meant to be. You aren't who you are right now. You are only what society has created you to be." From that day on, I sat back and thought about everything that challenged me in life. I then realized that the things that happened to me weren't my fault, and it was time to ask for forgiveness. I wanted to truly forgive those who made me *Believe* that I was worthless, nothing other than a punching bag to be knocked down and made to feel as if I had nothing to offer this world. Just like some women, I always knew there was so much more to me inside, but I never allowed it to shine.

    Once I identified why I allowed the vibrant, healthy me to vanish, I finally exhaled and was able to breathe once again. Armando, you saw something in me that I didn't. Like you always say, it's not you, Armando, who saved me. It was me who heard the truth, and it's me who saved myself. You guided me to learn about myself and to find that person who was within. Once I grasped hold of that, the more I was feeling better about myself internally and externally. Through simple gradual progression the pounds began to come off, and the days were being filled with signs and that of joy. I didn't struggle with finding who I was because I understood that these life circumstances were now nothing but life lessons, and I knew that I had to be aware of what's around me. If I noticed someone acting a certain way, I knew not to move forward down that path. If I felt my pants getting tighter, I never needed to get on a scale. I knew that I needed to assess what it was that I ate that week and learn from it. There's so much more to life than feeling uncomfortable in your own skin, and that's definitely no way to live.

God gave me a life, a life that I was meant to live. I was not meant to let someone else control my life for me—not food or alcohol or a person telling me what I can or cannot do. Years of my life were ripped away from me, and I had a choice. I could have continued living life this way or take hold of it. I chose to make my life my own. Not in a selfish way but living life!!! Now I smile every day, I am energetic, I love my family and friends, and I give to others all the love that I know is inside of me.

So, as I sit here and reflect on everything that I had gone through and where I am today, the feelings that I feel within cannot be expressed. It's funny because when I was depressed, I always wrote about those feelings or, like most women, would turn to a friend to complain about the negatives in life. But now that I am on my way to living a life of complete joy and happiness, pain free, free of anger, hurt or deceit, I don't see the negative. My happiness is a feeling I have within, and guess what? Those people around me feel what I felt from you when I first met you. That energy!!! The way I feel on a regular basis is absolutely priceless. I am the woman I was meant to be.

What woman or person for that matter wouldn't want to live life like mine on a daily basis?

Tears once again roll down my cheeks because you are in my life—tears of joy. I can't thank you enough for seeing that there was so much more to me than just someone coming to train with you. If I could stand on top of a mountain and scream your name for the world to hear, I would because your guidance and wisdom is what this world is missing in order to be a happier place to live. A gift from God had been sent to me, one that I didn't overlook, one that I didn't take advantage of, one that I didn't just say I want to lose 30 pounds and move on with my life. That gift was you and your guidance.

You are wise with your words, caring, joyful, and an amazing individual! You live the life most often dream of...like a fairytale, a fairytale that I now know I can live too because I *Believe*! With living this way, I know that the energy I feed off will bring a beautiful man in my life to live happily ever after with and create the family that I had always dreamed of having.

Keep living your dream! Have faith! And *Believe* that you are going to be successful with the goals you have recently set for yourself! Remember, and I said it, there's a whole world out there, and it needs you!

I'm here for you, under your tent, to follow in your footsteps and make dreams become reality! "Together we can accomplish the unimaginable" ~Armando Aversa.

You rock! You're the best! I'm so lucky to have you in my life :)

Thank you!!!!

Michelle

"In a world where you can be anything, be yourself!"
—Etta Turner

I figured Michelle was the perfect candidate and the perfect person to walk with me on the next part of my journey; so I offered her the experience of putting together this book with me and head all of the marketing and sales. She was ecstatic, and sure enough she said yes. She believed!

I informed her we would leave the following morning. She asked, "Why not today?" She was eager to begin. I said, "Something is telling me to leave tomorrow morning." She smiled.

As we drove to Newport, I began entertaining another feeling, a burning, immense feeling—similar to the rush of emotion I felt in Dallas but undefined. As we approached Newport, rather than going directly to the house, I felt compelled to take Michelle to a specific spot I enjoyed a few years earlier along The Cliff Walk.

I took a right hand turn on Ocean Drive, which is a canopy road embraced by flowering trees, a sinuous road that takes one directly to an entranceway on The Cliff Walk.

As soon as I turned right, the sun aligned perfectly with the road. The heat from the sun penetrated the front windshield and swept over us. I felt suddenly bathed in brilliance and goodness, much as I had felt that morning in Dallas. The sign felt unmistakable. Understanding and wisdom suffused me. I felt lighter, more free, and more thankful than ever before in my life. The pieces came together. I saw for the first time the whole picture, the entire design, the unmistakable pattern of my belief and truth.

Michelle felt the rush of meaning, too.

I said to Michelle, "Wow, if that's not a sign, what is?"

She was speechless and in awe, smiling as the radiance lit her features.

I pulled the truck to the side of the road and jumped out to take pictures. I stood in the middle of the road and embraced the rays of sun on my face. Not one car appeared to interrupt my feeling as I stood in the middle of the road.

After a few moments of reveling in the glory of the site, we got back in the truck and continued to drive, full of wonder. The sun guided us to the end of the road, directly to my favorite spot. I gathered my backpack, headphones, iPod, and my tape recorder. I turned to Michelle: "I'll call you when I'm done." I walked toward the sun and down a rocky path.

The view was majestic. The sun hung over the crystal water. There was no one to interrupt my thoughts, and an energy flowed through me that felt boundless. I looked at the ocean and put my iPod on and continued to walk. I soon realized the music was a distraction; I shut it off and sat in silence. The coastline was amazingly peaceful. I lay on a flat rock with my eyes closed; no thoughts were coming to me. I didn't know where to start. My mind was completely empty. I embraced the moment fully, realizing I was given a blank piece of paper, and so I just lay in silence and patiently waited. I just knew my answers of truth would soon become clear. The sun snuck behind a cloud, and then at the perfect moment the light emerged.

Once again, I felt a sensation take over my thoughts. How is it possible that the weight loss approach I use has had such an impact on people's lives? The truth is deeper and far greater than looking and feeling better, far greater than fitting into sizes from college years.

Over the years of searching for the secret to weight loss, I have grown extremely empathetic. Over time, my empathy became a learned behavior that I worked on day in and day out. I became a person who could relate to others' feelings of pain and struggle. I guess my responsiveness arises from over 30,000 hours of conversations with women of all ages, shapes, sizes, and backgrounds. Think about this for a second. Imagine being a trainer 8 to 10 hours a day for close to 10 years, training women of all types. Imagine the variety and amount of conversations I shared and what I have learned from each person. I have gained wisdom that no one could pay for.

I could write a book about the best bras, underwear, or haircuts, colors and fashions—just imagine how many menstrual cycles I have experienced! I feel as if I have also gone through menopause! I've lived through pregnancies, miscarriages, breakups, divorces, good moods, bad moods, and crazy moods. I've been a best friend and a shoulder to cry on, and eventually I evolved into a great advice giver. I'm a pretty manly guy, but I have developed a very acute sensitivity to women, women's needs, and the pressures our culture places on women. Even with all the pressures and struggles women face, I still *Believe* they are the ones who will tackle adult and childhood obesity.

I became familiar and sensitive to my clients, living and learning through their experiences, embracing what others go through in relationships, parenting, and struggles with eating. Their stories inspired my passion to grow even more toward finding an approach to encourage weight loss. I wish everyone a better life, and if I can be part of guiding someone down the right path, then I have fulfilled part of my destiny. Life is far too beautiful not to live in joy and peace—and far too precious not to use one's gifts and talents.

Along with being empathetic, I also tapped into being extremely intuitive. We all share an ability to trust our instincts. However, it is up to the individual to connect to his or her soul. If I had not matured my ability to act intuitively, I would not have been led to Dallas or to Newport. Without those journeys, this book would not exist. We can find balance in our lives and trust what we think and feel.

I'm confident there are times in your life when you feel empathetic and/or intuitive. Sometimes, we fail to heed our intuition or ignore our realization; I know I have, and I'm guessing there are times when you haven't trusted your instincts and wished later you had. We were all born with the specific gift of intuition. That gift will assist you in reaching your goals and divine destiny. Your intuitiveness is what can guide you throughout your life. Growing your empathetic nature will provide you the shared feelings of others. We gain our instincts and wisdom by carefully watching ourselves and others, by simply seeking and acknowledging the truth.

You without question can tap in to your intuitive mind; your mind is rich with endless guidance and wisdom. With the right foundation, being still and sitting in silence will work wonders in your quest for your truth.

While sitting on The Cliff, I recorded hours of thoughts that surfaced from deep within my subconscious, thoughts that were once again from my soul. After hours of speaking into the recorder, I thought, Why me? How is it possible that I have the cure for weight loss? There has to be a reason why I was chosen. I didn't feel special, and I didn't have an answer that made sense to me, so I continued speaking into the recorder for another hour.

One of the many thoughts I recorded was my impression of how I grew as a trainer. I developed my approach by learning from others, by seeking the depths of those who don't succeed and those who do, those who lost weight but still struggled keeping it off and those who just didn't want to hear the truth. When it comes to weight loss and life, success depends on learning from our mistakes, setbacks, troubles, and failures. Mistakes and setbacks are successes when one learns from them. Acknowledging this truth will lead to success. Without tough times, we wouldn't grow and evolve into our more perfect, fully realized selves. I'm not saying we need tragedy in our lives, but when obstacles appear, going through them and not around them is a must. The more people try to dodge obstacles the more the obstacles will reappear.

With weight loss, this is the common theme: follow this diet, do this program, try this system. When it's all said and done, most are standing with their hands in the air, time wasted and pockets emptied. One of the biggest mistakes one can make with weight loss and life is not looking at these moments of anxiety, despair, and difficulty as opportunities for growth. If you are overweight and upset, now's your chance to grasp the truth; you will feel a sense of empowerment far greater than any diet could ever offer, and your anger will disappear.

There are only two ways to grow and evolve. One is learning from our mistakes. The other is hearing and embracing the truth. For some, a few attempts at acknowledging the truth may be necessary to come to a realization. For others, embracing the truth may happen within the moment of hearing it. Regardless, the most important element is, eventually believing in the truth. Perhaps we don't need a mistake or setback or trouble to inspire us to grow and evolve. However, if one deals with an obstacle, makes a mistake, or has a setback, one has the opportunity for transformation. In a sense, hardship can be used as a blessing. Or is hardship a blessing in disguise?

The most successful people in the world use failures, mistakes, and setbacks as opportunities to create success in the future. Often, our failures are springboards to living a better life. Those who embrace the possibility of transformation from failure evolve and succeed. Those who don't continue to spin their wheels and live life as the majority of those in society do, aimlessly searching for the answers, the easy way, or a quick fix. Many false paths might seem like the easy way, but hearing and embracing the truth will ultimately be the most rewarding way to success and happiness! It's the only way!

I have made my share of mistakes, some I wish I could take back. I have regretted the consequences of some of my poor choices, but I don't *Believe* ignoring or forgetting my mistakes is useful. Why? When temptation strikes in the future, I use the feelings I have embraced in troubled times to overcome any weakness or vulnerable moments. Success lies with how one learns from mistakes, not by forgetting about them. We must ingest the horrible feelings that come from hurting others or ourselves to avoid them later. If we don't embrace the uncomfortable feelings that attend horrible choices, and we sweep them under a rug as if they never happened; sooner or later, we'll have to deal with the dirt, and our life is full of lumps. I choose always to remember not to punish myself but to know I would attempt to never repeat my once destructive actions. It is important to embrace the negative feelings that come with binge eating, overindulging, and poor food choices.

For example, when someone is eating healthy and that person decides to indulge in old, unhealthy habits (say some fried foods, a couple of candy bars, or one too many trips to the buffet), no doubt a stomach ache will afflict them. And I don't mean an emotional belly ache from feeling guilt; no, your body will rebel, and you will pay a physical price. You may not pay much attention to the feeling at first, but don't worry, your subconscious is making a list. Even better, make the feeling conscious—make the direct connection between eating poorly and feeling poorly, and then you can change the habit. The next time you want an extra scoop of ice cream, remember the belly ache and you will indulge less.

We can become conscious of the positive feelings, too—in fact, being aware of and grateful for how good we feel when we are healthy is essential. After a healthy meal, a fresh walk, a good conversation, we will feel alive and happy: store those feelings in your conscious memory so that they will become a positive, habitual presence in your life.

We will all face temptations as we try to lose weight, but realizing we can learn from our poor choices when temptation strikes, that we can use our mistakes as a lesson that teaches us to avoid repeating them, is tremendously empowering. We cannot hide from temptations; ultimately, we have to overcome them, and with the truth as a foundation, we will!

From a training standpoint, I have made my share of mistakes as well—like putting clients on diets and programs. My commitment to these fads was very short lived because I saw within my first year of training clients ten years ago, that these programs were an approach that simply don't work long term. Look in any bookstore, and you'll see plenty of books offering many great approaches, but nothing works 100% of the time for every individual. I'm not putting a theory together that works for some on a short term. I want everyone to be successful 100% of the time, long term, effortlessly, and with an outcome greater than just losing weight and looking good. I want people to see the light at their own feet, to accomplish the weight loss they have tried to achieve their whole life themselves.

In the course of my progress, I examined all the other approaches in an effort to find the ultimate answer: how do we lose and keep weight off? By constantly learning and evolving, I arrived at the truth about how to lose weight.

Your way is the only way.

After I confirmed my realization, I decided in the second half of my training days never to put a client on a diet or program. I've simply guided them with thoughts and ideas. I never preached to my clients; we just shared conversations. I answered questions based on fact and truth.

Only those who heard the truth were successful; those who sought their truths and learned from their daily occurrences succeeded 100% of the time.

The magnitude of what I have learned is beyond priceless. For my own personal life, for what I do as a career, and for the hundreds of millions in search for the answer to weight loss, one truth exists for your success.

As I sat on the rocks fully engulfed in the moment, my subconscious took me back to numerous times in my life when I could see things happening before they did. I'm not claiming to be a psychic, but I am saying I have grown to be very connected to my inner soul. I had a feeling that my weight loss approach was the reason I felt this connection although I just never could quite figure out exactly why. How is such prescience possible? Was it God? I always believed in God but it's not like at this time in my life that I was going to church often or even read the bible.

The waves crashed. The starlings cluttered the sky. I sat peacefully on The Cliff Walk. All of a sudden, my mind went blank. I enjoyed the stillness in the air and my mind; I rested in the great pleasure of being still. After five or ten minutes, I looked to see how long I had been talking into the recorder. I had recorded nearly two hours worth of thoughts and ideas. The words, the thoughts emerged from the depths of my soul, my subconscious mind.

They were mine, of course, but tethered to a deeper truth—one each of us contains although is up to us to fully access.

I called Michelle and asked her to pick me up. I walked back to the entrance and waited. She arrived, smiling as always.

"How did it go?" Michelle smiled at me, her hands on the steering wheel. "Incredible! A presence was there that words could never describe. What I was feeling and saying was so vivid, so true, and so real."

Michelle patted and squeezed my arm. "I want to hear!"

We drove to a spot on the beach because I wanted to capture the moment and possibly use a picture for the book. We took the picture, and as we were walking off the beach, I showed a complete stranger the picture of what I thought at the time was going to be the front cover of the book.

I said, "Look at this picture. Isn't it beautiful?"

"Remarkable," she said, taking a second look. "Are you a photographer?"

I told her I was a trainer and that I was writing a book. She asked me the name.

I hadn't thought of a title yet.

"*Believe,*" I said, surprised at my choice—and delighted. "I'm going to call the book *Believe*."

In a European, beautiful accent, she said, "I *Believe*."

I thanked her and walked away. The beach had given me clarity and a title. I asked for little, and the world gave back much.

Be Still.

~ Your Personal Notes ~

6.

After we arrived at our accommodations for the weekend, I noticed a book on the kitchen table. I asked Michelle about the book, and she informed me my father had given it to her to give to me.

"A book!" I picked it up. "Why in the world would my father be giving me a book? I've never read a book in my life. I got through college by listening attentively and skimming. Don't worry, I was a good student."

Michelle looked up from the magazine she was reading and said, "Perhaps it's time."

I smiled back at her.

I took the book with me and went upstairs. I thumbed through a few of the pages. I stopped on a random page. I don't know why I stopped, but I stopped when I felt as if I should. I couldn't *Believe* my eyes. Everything that I was reading was literally everything I was talking about on The Cliff. My hands began to shake.

And there it was…Boom! I had the answers to why I felt connected. What I spoke of on The Cliff was only part of the message. What I read seemed wise and knowledgeable. The words suggested experiences from our life that are far greater than the finest gold.

I could not *Believe* what I was reading.

I almost fainted. I couldn't *Believe* my good fortune. I realized I was on to something huge. All of the thoughts I spoke of on The Cliff were truth, and they were all in the book.

As I continued to read, the word "*Believe*" kept appearing. I was blown away with how many times I saw the word "*Believe*."

Another realization dawned: my discussion on the beach was no accident. The title of my book was no accident. **Life is**

bursting with possibilities and connections if we are willing to see and accept them.

I closed the book. I decided to continue with my journey, collecting my subconscious thoughts. I wanted *Believe* to be authentic and real. My father's book inspired another truth, and I was ready to move closer to my destiny and your answer to weight loss! I could have made quick correlations from the book to my life and taken an easy way out of my journey, but instead I continued forward. I don't *Believe* in shortcuts—the truth is always in the journey. It didn't feel right to stop searching. I trusted my instinct; I wanted my subconscious to guide me.

~ Your Personal Notes ~

7.

The book my father gave me generated an inspirational surge of energy and enthusiasm. My heart beat nearly out of my chest, pounding as if I had just won the lottery--and in a sense I had. I was closer to helping tens of millions lose weight, become healthy, and be happy, which in my mind is beyond priceless. Life is precious, and the lives of those who are struggling are as valuable as any. I was now close to fulfilling my passion to help tens of millions.

After a relaxing and wonderful weekend, Michelle and I packed and headed home. I felt completely peaceful. While I was driving, I decided to check my voicemail. I received a frantic phone call from my brother, Joe. I thought my house had blown up. I called him immediately and begged to know what was going on. He informed me my fish tank had leaked, and all the water traveled into the basement. He encouraged me to come home immediately.

I asked him how much damage was done. He considered for a moment and then said it wasn't so bad, especially considering how bad it could have been.

"Some of your basement ceiling tiles are ruined."

"Did any fish die?"

"No, they are all alive, but there is only a quarter of the water left in the tank."

My panic had already subsided, and Joe was beginning to calm down, too. I thanked him for the call and told him I would be home in a few hours and that I was already on my way. He said, "Really? That's a lucky coincidence."

I developed into a truly optimistic person. Rather than getting upset and ruining the mood I was in, I looked at the bright side. I had to change the water in the tank anyway. At least now, I didn't have to empty it. Seriously, if getting upset or frustrated helped the problem, then I would have punched the steering wheel a few times and done 100 mph all the way home. But why? What's the sense of getting frustrated or upset? The truth is, panicking and over-reacting doesn't make sense. Early in my life, a friend questioned me about my negativity and pessimistic ways. I have to say her questions shocked me; I never realized I was a pessimist. Luckily and thankfully, that friend had the courage to suggest my negative energy was not useful or attractive. She changed the course of my life. I'm grateful she told me and I heard the truth.

If we aren't vigilant, negativity can grab us, shake us, and force us to lose our perspective. The world is wonderful. We are wonderful. Accidents are part of a larger plan—a destiny that allows us to see sunshine even when there are clouds, to see advantages in situations that seem ruinous. Negative thoughts and behaviors can ruin a fantastic day—or a week, a month, a life.

Our world is stuffed full of pessimists, those who see the world as half ugly rather than all beautiful. Many of the same people perpetuate their pessimism with a self-pitying, "why me?" attitude.

Self-pity and pessimism will always undermine our desire to lose and keep weight off. Always! A negative attitude will make weight loss impossible, or if one does succeed, keeping the weight off will be a constant struggle and battle. Recognizing and abolishing our own pessimism is a difficult task even for the strongest; our world ingrains in us the right, the entitlement to complain and be negative. **To change, though, to fully accept the truth that negative thoughts lead to self destructive habits is an important step toward effective weight loss and living in the divine.**

I fully embraced my negativity when I was confronted and decided to continue to live my life and acknowledge each and every moment I was negative or pessimistic. Being consciously aware and acknowledging, and not overlooking, I was able to overcome. Such personal honesty and clarity seems daunting, but overtime, replacing the pessimism with the optimism, turning negative into positive, becomes habitual: it becomes you because being positive and optimistic is the type of attitude you were meant to have.

To lose weight, we must first transform our way of thinking. It takes looking at ourselves and our attitudes closely and recognizing the negative reactions that have so far ruled our actions. It doesn't need to be a difficult or hard truth to swallow. It is what it is and all that matters is realizing the truth to ones developed character flaws. Positive energy and outlook brings peace, peace brings happiness, and happiness leads to your success!

~ Your Personal Notes ~

8.

After I returned from Newport and cared for my fish, my life carried on as usual. I worked my typical 8 to 10 hour day training clients, collecting any thoughts that came to me during the sessions. And, of course, I continued to wake at the usual 3am to entertain thoughts that seemed to arrive out of nowhere.

As I was having breakfast one morning, I stared outside at my backyard in a daze. I was admiring the beauty of my property and all the remaining Christmas trees. I began to think how fortunate and grateful I am to have been given such a beautiful, flat, two acre piece of property. When I turned twenty-four, my father and mother approached me and offered me the family tree farm to manage and sell Christmas trees.

Yes, I was delighted and surprised, but at the time I also said to myself, what in the world am I going to do with a tree farm? Frankly, I wasn't quite sure what I'd do with a tree farm with over 1,000 Christmas trees. I assumed I'd play Santa Claus every Christmas. I worked diligently on the farm the next few years. I did enjoy seeing all the little kids run around picking out their tree and the physical labor of sawing and tying hundreds of trees each day in freezing temperatures. Walking through the trees on my property, enjoying the crisp weather and deep snow, I had the opportunity for my thoughts to swim around in my head. I often allowed ideas to pop in from strange angles.

One day, while watching a red-tailed hawk circle near the border of the trees, I had a sudden thought: I am going to build a home when I am twenty-eight. Why twenty-eight? Because something told me to. I'm not a big believer in setting times and dates for experiences that are out of my control. But building a house seemed real and possible. I felt compelled to build, like I had to. I wouldn't say I was Noah building an ark, but a similar inspiration, a similar directive, filled me with the desire to construct my home.

I visited my parents to share the news. When I told my father my plans to build a house when I turned twenty-eight, he said, "Are you crazy? Do you know how much money you need to build a house?"

He stared at me for a moment. I couldn't tell if he was genuinely disbelieving or intrigued by my sudden passion.

"You don't even know how to build a house."

I laughed and told him, "I know! But, I'll figure it out." I became serious. "Something told me that I'm going to build a house by the time I was twenty eight."

"Something? What do you mean, something?"

"I have no idea, Dad. Something. I don't know what to tell you. I'm going to build a house." We shared a look. "Don't worry. Everything will be fine."

His look told me he had sided with disbelief. He said, "Ok. Whatever you think."

I didn't blame my father for not believing my vision the same way I did because at the time he and I both knew I didn't make a lot of money, nowhere near enough to afford a mortgage let alone build a home.

Three years later when I was still making the same amount of money as I was at twenty-four, I knew I would be fine because I had a plan to start my own business. I had what felt like a million Christmas trees on two acres of property, and I thought, "What in the world am I going to do now?" I sold a bunch of trees every Christmas throughout the years, but a thousand or so trees remained on the land where I wanted to build the house. For a moment, I thought, this is impossible. I can't just cut them down. The waste would shock my brother and parents. I figured I could sell them next year and the years to come from out of my backyard, but I needed to get them there.

Transplanting a Christmas tree that's six, seven, eight feet tall could take anywhere from twenty to thirty or even forty minutes. If I was to tackle the project alone, I'd constantly be getting on and off the backhoe, trying to hold the tree up straight while I tried to dig it up out of the ground. If the tree fell over, I'd have to get off the machine to pick it back up. I saw an enormous amount of difficult labor ahead of me, but what choice did I have? I began the work.

The first few trees took me a great deal of time; I had difficulty keeping them straight, and the time necessary to do the labor of two or three men compounded the difficulty. Once I brought the tree over to its new home to a hole I previously dug, I had to attempt to place the tree in the hole; invariably, I'd watch it fall over, get out of the machine, stand it upright, try to wedge it upright, and fill dirt along the sides; then I had to pack the soil around the tree, water the tree, tamp the earth, straighten it, tie stakes to keep it straight, add more dirt, and re-water. I was a complete amateur, but I was earnest and dedicated. As the days progressed, I learned from my mistakes, and the work became easier—even enjoyable. I became a pro after the first three or so weeks.

During the first week, I felt the task was impossible. I almost quit. I figured I would have to wait to build the house until all the trees were sold. In between planting two trees, sitting on the backhoe, I thought to myself, if I keep moving a few each day, patiently tackling the job in increments, the work wouldn't be so bad and eventually all the trees would be transplanted. **Simple progression.** When I imagined the whole job, I felt overwhelmed; when I imagined how I could complete the work a little at a time, I didn't get overwhelmed. How long would the entire process take? I didn't focus on the question. I figured, as long as I am progressing toward my goal of moving a few each day, inevitably they will all be moved. I banished my thoughts that led to a feeling of being overwhelmed; I could easily handle two, three, or even four trees a day.

I enjoyed the small work of moving individual trees, so why allow the thought of moving a thousand trees to cause any anxiety? Why continue to count the remaining trees? A similar thought occurs to the majority who constantly weigh themselves rather than focusing on the task at hand. Such a focus on the scale just doesn't make sense. Trust me! With weight loss as with moving trees, all that truly matters is progress. With incremental progress, it's inevitable the results will come. The pounds will come off. They always do in time. How fast? Quick fixes are not the answer. You can, of course, get short term results from many diet shakes, meals, programs, or pills, but over time, 95% of these will fail, and the weight will return.

The work was difficult, certainly at first, but over the first weeks, my skill level increased dramatically because I learned as I went along and found ways to become more efficient. I was able to move more trees each day. Eventually, I succeeded at moving 10 to 20 trees a day.

Suddenly and without much real drama or trauma, all the trees were moved. The entire process took significantly less time and effort than expected. My original vision of the ordeal did not come to pass; once I chose to focus on the positive, smaller increments of work, I *Believe* moving the trees took four or five months. I did not mind the work; all that mattered to me was the daily progress, the thoughtful and steady application of work that resulted in my cleared land and the transplantation of nearly 400 trees I had moved just enough trees to build the house. I figured I would move the remaining trees, those in my immediate backyard, when the time was right.

I had real evidence now of something I've come to *Believe* and trust: when I have a good foundation, a goal, and when I take smaller, incremental, positive steps, success is guaranteed. And the same goes for weight loss. Losing weight comes down to **gradual, steady progression**. We don't need to move all the trees at once, and we don't need to lose all the weight—or change all of our habits—at once. One tree, one pound, one new way of thinking at a time and, suddenly, we're in a beautiful new house and a beautiful, healthy, revived, new you!

A scale to record our weight is only valuable when we've achieved our natural weight, the weight we were meant to be. Debbie was down to a size 6 after her amazing transformation from a snug 12. She then weighed herself and weighed 132 pounds. She was a little shocked. She thought she should be around 124 pounds. She looked like she weighed 120 and felt even thinner! But, she chose to trust the scale, which is a mistake. She was rid of all excess body fat and was her perfect size and weight. She now uses the scale daily or weekly to help measure her progress and maintenance. If she goes over 135, she knows she has fallen off track and has made either poor choices with her eating or exercise.

Once you have found your natural weight, a scale is useful to help you assess your fitness relative to that natural weight point. You can get on the scale if your pants feel a little snug or you're feeling a little sluggish—just to see your current weight. But the scale can't control you; your feelings of empowerment and health control your choices and decisions. The scale is only a small tool. Our bodies naturally fluctuate daily one to four pounds—so don't go crazy if you gain a pound or two.

Some days, I moved ten trees, and then I didn't move a single tree for days. Of course, I had plenty of trees remaining. Now suppose I allowed myself to be diverted from my task and made some poor choices. We all are prone to making poor choices once in a while. What if I waited long enough for a few new seedlings to sprout? Now I had even more trees to move! When one doesn't hide from the truth and learns from their poor choice that seedling can be easily moved within minutes. If one decides not to acknowledge and learn from a poor choice, that seedling will develop and root. It will grow and continue to grow and hinder me from achieving my goal. After a while, after I've hidden the truth from myself that new seedlings are sprouting, the day will arrive when I realize a new forest has appeared and all my earlier work will have to be repeated.

Those new, rooted trees will be difficult to move. The extra ten pounds you gained will be difficult to lose—a lot more difficult than the daily maintenance of eating well and exercising! One tree is easy to take out if we recognize that a tree has appeared. It's much easier to acknowledge the truth (of a poor choice or habit) and learn from a mistake than hiding from the consequences and allowing the situation to become worse.

And remember, having a dessert in moderation is not a mistake or poor choice. But living life hiding from our truths is!

~ Your Personal Notes ~

9.

In the weeks following my return from The Cliff Walk in Newport, I continued to work on my book, to record my thoughts, but I felt I was losing my inspiration. I questioned why I was writing a book and if I had the talent to finish the project. Writing is difficult work. I was concentrating on the larger project instead of the act of creation, the individual thoughts I was recording, and I began to lose sight of the joy the experience had been providing me. Don't think I don't struggle. Life is about overcoming these thoughts that try to sabotage our success. We can overcome the messages society portrays that divert us from the truth; we can overcome negative distractions.

Luckily, I am very aware of my surroundings because what happened during the next few weeks provided signs and guidance that eliminated permanently any doubt or questioning.

On two separate days, I was sitting in the backyard writing when I saw a white squirrel and a white rabbit. They both hopped around as if they hadn't a care in the world. They must have stayed in my yard for hours, playing and scavenging. Their robust activity was both entertaining and rejuvenating. I'd never seen a white rabbit and white squirrel; I didn't know if white squirrels or white rabbits were common in the wild, so I did a search online.

According to Answer Bag website (found at http://www.answerbag.com/q_view/116934), mysticstonecarver says, "A *white rabbit* often foretells the possibility of spiritual enlightenment and/or an encounter with the Divine. White rabbits are metaphors that signify an invitation to step out of ordinary time. If you see a white rabbit, you have been chosen; it is not necessary to know or to ponder why. They call us out from our ordinary life to go on an extraordinary journey that will lead us to a transformative experience. The white rabbit is an invitation. The rabbit never coerces but gently compels us to let go of what we think is important and to explore what is of ultimate importance. They are an invitation to enter the realm of the real, hidden, intuitive, unconscious world that exists underneath what appears to be reality. The unlikely pilgrim will be taken to places that she or he never dreamed possible and the passage will cost more than what most are willing to freely give. If you happen upon a white rabbit, remain awake and alert to the direction you must go and be ready to let go of everything you believed was important. You do have a choice. You can continue what you were doing and ignore the invitation. Your life will continue its placid, unenlightened course."

I felt a rush of inspiration. At the precise moment I felt a lag in my commitment to my goal, a lull in the desire to continue my book, when my faith started to waver, I ran across not one but two days of white rabbits. Faith was sent to me when I needed uplifting most.

According to Angels & Dragons & Fairies, Oh, My!, site (found at www.angelsdragonsfairies.com/animaltotem.htm), "the gathering power of a *squirrel* is a great gift. The animal's power teaches us balance within the circle of gathering and giving out."

Ah, balance—giving and taking: the other side of my inspiration! The squirrel reminded me that faith is given, that inspiration is divine, but that I can't only take: I have to give, too. Just as inspiration fills me, I must also fulfill my destiny to write and share the truth.

After my encounter with the white woodland creatures, my energy increased and I continued recording and writing out my thoughts. I was refreshed and invigorated.

A while later I shared a conversation with a close friend of mine about hummingbirds. She was saying how she loves hummingbirds and how amazing they are. I said, "Hummingbirds?" She mentioned that a variety of hummingbirds lived in Connecticut and was surprised I had never seen one. She thought I was joking. We teased a little back and forth, and then I said I would be more aware so I, too, could see a hummingbird.

After our conversation had ended, my friend left my house and I decided to make a sandwich (yes, I eat bread, and so can you; whole grain, of course ☺). As I ate, I walked around my house, ending finally at a picture window overlooking my backyard.

Within ten seconds of standing near the window, surveying the trees and the bright, sunlit sky, I saw in the distance something coming at the window that looked like a miniature missile.

A hummingbird. Yes, a shimmering green and blue hummingbird darted to the window at lightning speed, suspended itself in midair, seemed to stare at me, and then vanished. The encounter was brief—all hummingbird encounters are brief—but the impact of the little drop of magic's presence was profound, and I seemed to have him in my gaze for an eternity.

Of course, the coincidence startled me, but I was beginning to *Believe* there were no coincidences, that even the smallest, most delicate encounters combined to make a larger whole, a more profound meaning. The hummingbird's beautiful movements, the decisiveness of its flight, and the sincerity of its presence at the precise moment I wanted to see a hummingbird renewed my faith that the world is benevolent and joyful.

I finished my sandwich and searched the symbolism of hummingbirds.

According to Lynx Graywolf site (found at http://morningstar.netfirms.com/hummingbirdmedicine.html), "Blessed are *hummingbirds* and the people who carry their medicine. In the modern world, many people are seeking to reconnect with the old ways of being to heal the feelings of disconnection bubbling within them, their families, and all of life. Many in today's world feel isolated and alone, unsure of where their right place in life is or if they have a purpose for being here. When we tune into the energy of a Hummingbird, we soon find that all of us are here for a divine purpose, and that purpose is to help heal ourselves and the planet. Through joy we manifest value and meaning for us. Hummingbird teaches us how to protect the experiences that bring us joy and encourages us to feel happy. Hummingbird people teach the rest of us how to protect and respect experiences and encounters that provide value and meaning to our own lives; they banish anything or anyone who chooses to try and invade our own sacred space."

My thoughts began pouring into the tape recorder. Ideas emerged on paper. My inspiration continued for days. And then I had a dream of two beautiful, colorful birds flying over my house in slow motion. Every color seemed magnified, every movement enhanced. I couldn't remember having a similar dream. The next morning, the same friend came over and I told her about the crazy dream I had about these two amazing birds flying over my house.

She thought the dream must be a sign.

As we were talking, I glanced over her right shoulder, and in the window, two exotic guinea hens sat on the sill. My jaw must have dropped because she asked what was wrong. I took out my camera phone and said, Look. She couldn't *Believe* what we were both seeing.

We both smiled and enjoyed the moment. After we finished her session, I walked over to the computer and did a search.

According to Irene of Cyprus site, (found at http://www.guineafowl.com/fritsfarm/guineas/Eustolios), "*Guinea Hens* are indicative of a deep faith and devotion to Christianity."

The gorgeous hens affirmed what I already knew. For years, the signs had been manifesting in my life, the fog had been lifting; my faith, like the hens, perched quietly just outside the window, waiting for me to open the sash.

Signs present themselves to us daily and are all around us. We can learn to read them, can learn to be receptive to their messages. I *Believe* things do happen for a reason. I could have looked at these happenings as coincidences and in turn still felt an absence of faith. But I *Believe* all things are connected, so I acknowledged what was going on around me and did the research. I allowed the connections to become real to me. I read the signs. Do you *Believe* in signs? Are you aware of signs? Perhaps we all already *Believe* in signs, but some of us are still skeptical that signs are sent from above. Perhaps some of us *Believe* life's small intersections are mere accidents, mere coincidences. I *Believe* this picture will convince even the hardiest doubters. Even some of the most obvious signs can be overlooked or missed even for the better at times. Luckily, I eventually came across this sign in the sky, in the following picture that was taken along the journey:

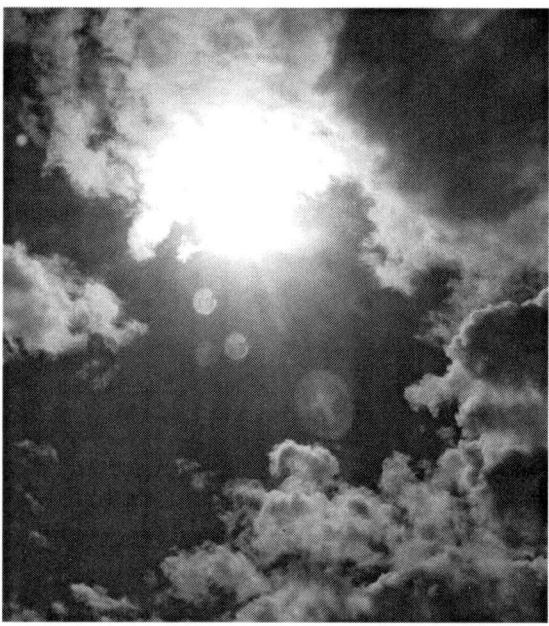

I had this picture on a calendar for numerous months until one day around the time of Newport I walked over and was flipping through and saw that cross in the sky. I was energized by what I saw and couldn't *Believe* the picture had hung in my office for a number of months, but I had never seen it, had never really paid attention to the picture. I saw the cross at a moment I needed inspiration, a time once again when I literally wanted to give up.

Realize that we are going to have down moments in our lives, but it's not a matter of how many times we get knocked down as long as we get up, learn, and move forward. At that moment, nothing was going to stop me from putting a book together. I felt energy surge through me. All the small work that seemed impossible or difficult had vanished. All the obstacles that appeared insurmountable seemed very small. With startling clarity, everything became apparent: the ideas surfacing from my subconscious could revolutionize the world and help conquer childhood and adult obesity.

Enjoy the beauty of your journey every moment of every day. The journey and the signs along the way will keep you inspired—not just the end goal. What happens along the way, the small miracles of white squirrels, hummingbirds, crosses in the sky are as priceless as reaching the goal. We should make efforts **to become aware**, in tune to God's messages and signs, and to God's beauty. Without awareness, one can miss daily happenings that are worth just as much as reaching any goal. A beautiful life is stuffed full of small joys, that feeling that you can't wait to go to bed because you are anxious to see what the next day brings.

Whatever the next day brings—signs, feelings, troubles: each day is full of purpose and reason. That's the beauty of believing. Nothing gets in our way; anything that challenges us, contradicts our plans, or confuses us provides an opportunity for growth, an inspiring sign, or a beautiful moment.

Faith is a key component to weight loss. As individuals, we can become aware and receptive—we can see connections and allow joy into our lives. God provides the road signs; it is up to us to *Believe* in our destiny and follow them. God already knows what you truly need to know. We acknowledge our weaknesses and ask God for guidance. We just simply need to be aware and prepared to receive an answer to what we really need to know.

Be receptive and be open because only God knows what's best for you. What you may ask for and think you need to know might not be what God thinks is important for you at that particular moment. You can be receptive to all the miracles God provides as guidance without worrying about making a mistake or missing a sign because God will never give up on you. He will always work miracles in your life when you acknowledge the truth. There were many moments I felt down or defeated, but when you have faith and a strong belief, the consequences of negative occurrences are short lived because you see them as opportunities for growth since you know you are traveling down the road of truth.

~ Your Personal Notes ~

10.

I decided to travel to the Bahamas. I called Michelle to tell her of my plans, and she said, "Let me guess." I could feel her smiling. "You just felt like that's where you needed to go."

I said, "Yes. I mean, come on, the Bahamas?"

Going away by myself would be a first. Going to a foreign place without knowing anyone left me feeling somewhat uncomfortable although I knew it was going to be an interesting trip. I had a premonition that the experience would be transformative.

On a cold, snowy February day in Connecticut, I began my research for my trip to the Bahamas. I spoke to a representative who explored all sorts of options. A lot of places were booked or out of my price range. The agent offered other island vacations, but I was persistent; I intended to go to the Bahamas. Finally, he found an all-inclusive resort that had availability. I booked the trip, and a few weeks later I was off to the Bahamas.

I didn't know where I was going. I took the first place available within my price range. As I packed the day before my trip, I said to myself, wait a minute, I am going to the Bahamas by myself to write a book. Why does this feel so right but yet so weird?

I didn't have a publishing deal. I'd never written a book. I was traveling alone. My friends thought I might be a little crazy. I was taking a risk, I guess, but the trip never felt risky; I felt destined to write *Believe*, and I didn't doubt any of the steps along the way. A publisher would come when I needed one. *Believe* would find its way into book form.

Perhaps my choice to travel and write was bold; I never considered the journey dangerous or risky because I believed in my destiny, because I was taking joy with each little step, because I knew the thoughts I had were real and that I must share them. I believed in myself and my dreams; I had faith in my destiny and the signs I was witnessing. I believed in the truth!

Believe in yourself. No matter who is reading this, you can overcome any habit that has caused weight gain and develop a habit conducive to weight loss. *Believe*!

My journey illustrates the power of believing. And yours will as well!

My intuition was kicking in again. I felt like I was supposed to go. I knew I had to continue my journey to find the answers. I had to continue to seek the truth and trust my instincts.

No set dates and deadlines. No artificial organization or plan.

The flight to the Bahamas was unexceptional. I recall the pilot welcoming us to the island, relating the record low temps in the evening and highs during the day of sixty seven with a chance of rain.

While at customs I had to fill out a questionnaire one of the questions was, "Where did you purchase your ticket?"

I noticed that my ticket receipt said Doylestown, Pennsylvania. I had never heard of Doylestown; I assumed the travel agent's office was there. I laughed because my friend Jon's last name is Doyle. Jon's ambition, passion, dedication, and success is what drove me to search for my passion and purpose. He has been a major factor in my success. I found it fitting that his name would be spoken when I arrived. I knew with certainty, again, that I was heading in the right direction.

When I boarded the shuttle, only one other person was riding with me. I felt a little awkward, knowing I was traveling for business when most others were coming for pleasure. But I knew, too, that my business was going to be pleasant. I wanted to write.

He was by himself as well. He asked the typical questions. I told him I was writing a book. He asked who was going to publish it. I really didn't want to have the same conversation I had with my friends, but I grinned and said, "I'm writing without a publisher—so far."

"You mean you came all the way to the Bahamas to write a book and you don't have a publisher? Brash move."

"Maybe," I said. "But I'll get a publisher when I'm supposed to."

"You must *Believe* in what you're writing." We were looking out of the windows now, feasting on the lush vegetation and tropical blue sky.

"In fact," I said, "that's the title: *Believe*" to which he smiled and raised his eyebrows in shock.

He turned to smile at me. We talked about the book the rest of the way to the hotel. He was in awe of the theory and suggested I had a best seller on my hands. He wished me the best of luck. We shook hands and said goodbye.

Five months later, I had a friend request on *Facebook* from him. Our discussion, and my approach to weight loss, had stuck with him, and he had lost over 30 pounds since his trip. He only heard a skeleton of the idea.

In the Bahamas, when I first arrived at the hotel, I walked directly to my room. I opened the door and noticed the room was dark. Two of the lamps had burned out bulbs. The pictures on the wall were crooked by about seven inches. The room was comically in disarray. I had a choice: I chose to smile, straighten the pictures, and be thankful I was in the Bahamas embarking on an epic journey to write a book that would transform the lives of millions.

The next morning, I woke eager and excited, ready to begin writing. I wanted a little breakfast, a little island food to sustain me in my endeavors. I headed to the hotel restaurant. I am not a picky eater. I grew up in an Italian household where I ate whatever was on my plate, whatever my mother or father prepared for the day. Luckily, my parents always offered me the majority of our food from the land: vegetables, meats, fruit, and occasional pastries or sweets around the holidays. In the restaurant at the hotel, though, I faced an astonishingly unappetizing meal: the oatmeal was runny, the milk tasted like spoiled water, the coffee ran like mud, and the eggs were runnier than the oatmeal. I picked at the offerings, struggling to find something I could eat; I finally selected some fruit, a piece of ham, and a slice of whole grain toast.

As I sat in an unbalanced chair at a table that needed to be wiped, encouraging myself to think positively, I reflected on times I've gained weight in the past: I typically struggled with weight gain only during winter months. When I was conscientious, I could lose weight, but I always seemed to regain what I'd lost, and sometimes I'd gain more. Winters were always tough for me. I'd gain 10 to 15 pounds during the cold season. And on vacations: I would over-indulge at the buffets, eating ravenously whatever was placed in front of me. Sometimes, I wasn't even hungry, but I would eat, and then I'd overeat. I was eating mindlessly, eating to fill voids of winter depression.

On vacations, I used to feel I was obligated to eat as much as possible to get my money's worth, and I felt as if eating would make for a better vacation. That particular mindset meant, ultimately, that I was paying to put on 5 to 10 pounds of fat and feel horrible physically by the end of every vacation. I equated over indulgence with happiness on vacation. I talked myself into over eating; I found a justification. Although, it simply doesn't make sense when you really think about. It's all temporary satisfaction.

I didn't need a real answer even though I knew exactly where my over-eating would take me—to pounds and pounds of fat and a negative outlook and feeling. I used to *Believe* the sugary taste of unhealthy food was delicious, but is the taste really worth the extra calories or is the taste not even that good in the first place? I've learned that the healthier I eat, the tastier the healthy food is!

I had many excuses, many ways to perpetuate the cycle of weight gain, depression, sporadic weight loss, and weight gain, but it isn't a pleasant way to live. Why during the winter did I over eat? Because I was bored or because I became depressed due to the lack of sun and vitamin D? Perhaps. More likely, I maintained a negative attitude that prevented me from seeing the truth, from accessing the part of myself that reoriented me to a positive attitude.

We don't have to over-eat to enjoy a vacation, and we don't have to gain body fat because the winter blues have us down. What do we need? A new pattern of thinking, a new way of enjoying the world in all of its manifestations—a way to stop using food to fill a void that would be better filled with energy, desire, and a sense of joyful purpose.

Early in my life, I perpetuated a habit of doing something that doesn't help the situation but only masks my unhappiness momentarily. Food does taste good when we're bored; ice cream, a whole quart, will temporarily provide relief from a broken heart—but only momentarily! When I overate, I always became more depressed and, consequently, gained more weight. Luckily for me, I never allowed myself to gain more than 15 pounds, and I always lost the extra pounds by the spring. This year was going to be different. Gaining and losing weight just doesn't make sense, and the unhealthy feelings associated with gaining weight inhibited my more positive emotions. No food tastes as good as being lean and healthy feels. Our society sends us wrong messages—that we should indulge, eat what we want, and that exercise is too strenuous. Obviously, those messages are false. Eating healthy foods and staying physically active are key components to a happy, vibrant life!

I didn't need a different kind of ice cream or a new fruity drink; I needed a totally new perspective and outlook. I needed a new habit. I needed, finally, a behavioral thought change, an attitude I could acknowledge and make real. The truth.

I poked the runny eggs. No overindulging at this all inclusive.

After breakfast, I grabbed some extra fruit, some bottled water, my recorder, and a flip cam and headed to the beach.

As I walked to the beach, I saw a man in his early 40's doing push-ups. He performed them with the typical, gym-inspired technique—not wrong, exactly, but not maximizing the exercise with perfect form. I asked him if he would mind if I showed him something that would help him get more out of the exercise.

He said sure. He seemed puzzled at first until he tried the exercise again with a few adjustments to his form. He couldn't *Believe* the difference. He was blown away.

"I've been doing it wrong all these years," he said, bewildered.

"Not wrong," I offered, "just not 100% correct. You are now going to get more out of each rep and set and in turn better results."

"Oh, so I was doing it wrong." We both laughed.

"Who cares? At least now you know."

He thought for a moment. "Could you help me with some other exercises?"

I asked him if he did squats, and he said, "Yes, but they hurt my knees." I asked him to show me how he does them. I had no difficulty spotting the break in good form that caused his pain. I showed him the correct way to perform squats without hurting his knees, and then I demonstrated some other common exercises.

He was taken aback by how amazing it felt by making minor adjustments to his form. We ended up talking about his life on the island and about his belief in the importance of taking care of his body and his mind. I asked him his age; he was fifty-one. I complimented him on how young he looked and what great shape he was in. "I thought you were in your early forties, at most," I said. "Imagine, if you didn't waste your time all these years with imperfect form, I would have thought you were in your thirties!"

He laughed and patted me on the back. "Do most people perform exercises incorrectly?"

"Ninety-nine percent," I said, "Unfortunately. Most people could enhance their form. It's not so much that people are exercising wrong. It's just that we can get so much more out of each and every exercise just like you have."

He shook his head. "I'm grateful, my friend. Thank you!" I looked at him and said "You're very welcome. Give me your address and I will send you a copy of a DVD I am going to put together once my book is finished." He offered me a firm, hearty handshake.

I continued my walk to the beach. I realized that attitude is a lot like exercise; a small change in how we orient ourselves to the world and especially toward our place in the world could have dramatic results. It isn't as if we're all living wrong, but rather that we could all make minor adjustment to our attitude and achieve a great deal more, be significantly happier, and generally delight in the miracle of living a wonderful life. I also thought about how often I hear people say how difficult it is to change when it actually isn't at all. People who think it's difficult tend to misunderstand where their habits came from in the first place: they made them! We make habits—whether they are good or bad depends on how consciously aware we are to them. Changing for the better will only make life more enjoyable and prosperous. And much easier. We can tackle obstacles much easier with a positive attitude. Negative attitudes and bad habits always increase the difficulty of living happily and achieving goals. Always!

Good habits and a positive mindset equate to weight loss and a happier, more fruitful life. Think about this for a minute. Very true, isn't it?

~ Your Personal Notes ~

11.

That evening, I ventured to the main lobby where a television glowed between two potted ferns. The news was on. A massive snow storm was ravaging Pennsylvania. Take a guess what city?

Doylestown.

Are you kidding? I said to myself. I had never heard of Doylestown, but after I arrived in the Bahamas, suddenly the town was part of my larger consciousness.

My spirits were emboldened. Even such a small occurrence, that on the surface seems coincidental, confirmed my attitude and my choice. I was in the right place doing the right thing. I had great instincts as we all do, as always I continued to pay attention to them.

The night was surprisingly cold, freezing actually, so I headed back to the room to warm-up. Once in the room, I walked over to the thermostat and, to my surprise, discovered there was no heat! I remained calm and said to myself, no worries! I'll take a nice, hot shower, and when I get out, I will put on sweatpants and the long-sleeved shirt I brought. Unfortunately, even after I cranked the handle to full open, I couldn't get any hot water to come out of the shower! I calmly walked over to the phone and called the front desk. The man at the front desk was pleasant and apologized for the inconvenience and informed me the boiler had malfunctioned, probably because of the extreme cold. He reminded me the temperatures were the coldest in many years. The hot water would be turned back on as soon as possible.

Two days later, we had hot water.

Despite the inconvenience, which could have affected my mood, I enjoyed a productive two days. I was in the Bahamas to write a best seller. I oriented myself to the positive elements of my visit: the beautiful country, the friendly people, the peace of being alone, and the feeling that I had a purpose: all kept me motivated.

I tried to get some words on paper that first evening, but they felt forced rather than natural, so I decided to go to bed early. I would seek a fresh start in the morning after allowing my subconscious to rejuvenate.

I woke up early and decided to go see the sunrise. I felt relaxed and peaceful. My solitary walk felt empowering. I love people, and I'm a social, friendly person, but walking on the beach as the sun crested the flat, calm water, illuminating the palm trees behind me, was an astonishing feeling. I felt fully immersed in the moment: I wasn't worried about the past; I wasn't anxious about the future. I felt whole—me, the water, the trees, and the sun.

I sat in the sand and allowed my great luck to fully absorb me. After a while, when I got hungry, I ate a piece of fruit I had brought with me. When others started to appear on the beach, I decided to venture down the strip of sand. I walked for an hour. I spent the time reminiscing about life. As I surveyed the landscape, I began to think of all the wonderful, important people I have encountered in my life and during this journey. I felt exceptionally grateful and appreciative of past encounters with others. Each person I've met has been a gift to me. How often do people come in and out of our lives? How often do we realize there might be a reason? A purpose?

The concession stand was about to open as I returned; the fruit was delicious, but I was still hungry. I had to see what they offered. Burgers, fries, fried chicken fingers, and four types of liquors (they had run out of beer!). I ordered a hamburger and fries. I walked over to one of the natives on the beach selling sunglasses and said, "What's up, bro? You want to split this with me?" He said, "Yaaaa, man."

We enjoyed our lunch, chatting about the beauty of life and his life on the beach. We discussed how fortunate and blessed we are to be able to walk, talk, and eat good food to fuel our bodies. He began talking about how people develop a way of life or habit of eating more than one truly needs to live and be satisfied. Some don't even realize they've become addicted to having sweets every day or foods that are high in fat, fried, and loaded with unhealthy carbohydrates.

The satisfaction one receives from eating unhealthy foods is only momentary. The brief sense that the food tastes good is the only benefit! The only way to enhance this benefit and feeling is either eating more per meal or eating these types of foods more frequently. Therefore, people create a habit where they constantly have to have unhealthy food to achieve a similar satisfaction. The sweet taste of sugar is nice for a moment, but we need more and more sugar, more and more unhealthy food, to sustain the sensation.

When you eat healthy and in turn become lean, you feel better than any food that is unhealthy for you tastes.

I said, "Dude, I was just thinking about that earlier." When you eat healthy foods and feel healthy, you feel great every moment, every day of your entire life. So why would anyone want to eat unhealthy foods on a regular basis when the only benefit is momentary satisfaction? People think they are deprived when they eat only healthy foods (or on a diet), but really those who eat junk daily are depriving themselves of their health and life. We can eat whatever we want, but there are always consequences—good or bad. Sweets are not wicked; too many sweets daily have negative health consequences. We need to be moderate in our tastes. The danger is that we create habits of eating and over eating junk food when we should create habits of eating healthy food with junk food available to us when we really want it. And, after eating healthily for a while, the times one wants sweets are few and far between.

When one transforms bad habits into a healthier lifestyle, those foods that one once subsisted on, but that were unhealthy, actually taste better: a piece of cake every now and then is very delicious! There is the reward. Transforming your habits is not about never eating junk, but about unhealthy foods being the exception rather than the habit.

He looked at me in complete shock as we shared this similar thought and said, "Ya, man, that makes complete sense."

We continued eating and laughed as we fought over the last fry! I got it by the way. He asked me about my hobbies and how I spent my time in Connecticut. "I just live life fully," I said. I told him I enjoyed golf and fishing, motocross, snowmobiling, boating, and just lounging around. "I'm usually down to do anything," I said. I try not to set plans if I don't have to and leave myself open for what life brings my way.

"You sound like you have an interesting life, man," he said.

"Every day bro—I have a very exciting life!" Just because I'm healthy and have a spiritual faith, my life is definitely not boring. A good life is really about following our passions and utilizing our gifts and talents, not necessarily about doing thousands of small activities just to entertain ourselves. I could easily overindulge inappropriately—eating the wrong kinds of food, spending money lavishly, lazing around on the couch—but I would rather enjoy the simpler pleasures that surround me everyday—my hobbies, my passions. One can find great pleasure decorating a home, flying kites with children in the park, or making a nutritious meal for one's family. We don't need fancy; we don't need "over-the-top." We are fortunate to have a world filled brimming with daily joys. If one truly has gratitude toward a beautiful home, a nice car or stylish hair, so be it. Gratitude is key!

After our great discussion, I carried on with my day. We had enough food to sustain us and enough companionship to inspire us. Sharing a meal serves us in two important ways! Try it sometime. Whether it's with someone or you save half of your meal for later in the day. It works! Half a banana, apple, or a few grapes can hold you over to the next meal before you become ravenous and in turn, overeat.

A storm buffeted the island later that day. Gusts of 20 to 35 mile-per-hour winds rocked the windows, the temperature dropped precipitously, and the rain fell in massive sheets, often hurling sideways. I spent the majority of the afternoon in my room with no hot water, static on the TV, no heat, and the crooked paintings that I returned to their crooked position because I thought their off-square angles created comical relief.

During the storm, I enjoyed a magnificent view of the ocean. I could have despaired—being forced inside during my stay in the Bahamas—but when I closed my eyes and listened to the wind, when I focused on the sound of the palm trees creaking as they swayed, the rain pelting the window, the white caps marking the choppy surf of the ocean—I felt fortunate to be part of such a mystical, mysterious, wondrous world.

I had my tape recorder and writing material and the book my father had given me, but I didn't open them. I wanted to write, but the moment felt forced, and every time I put pen to paper, the words felt untrue. I needed to stay in my moment. Earlier in my life, I would have attempted to work my way through whatever was blocking me; I would have forced the issue and produced bad work, uninspired work. I've learned that I work best when I allow myself to feel the right moment, to feel and know when the time is right. How often do people try to force things to happen?

As I enjoyed the storm, my fingers casually manipulated my father's gift. I opened and closed the book randomly, not paying attention. After a while, I noticed I had been opening the book to a certain page, and so I turned to read. I wondered if I would find inspiration, if there would exist a correlation between my thoughts these past months and what I was experiencing now.

What I read startled and delighted me. The page contained several thoughts that echoed my sentiments about weight loss. My spirits were lifted. I shut the book and knew even more amazing insight would come from this trip. My vacation wasn't over. I still had two days left. I remained patient. As the sky darkened, the storm began to abate. The rain fell more gently, and the wind lessened. Perhaps I would be able to see stars later.

As I prepared for bed, I reflected on the strangeness of my trip so far. The cold weather, the cold showers, the runny eggs, and the crooked paintings: the adventure seemed more comical than divine. I wondered, was the vacation a test? I wonder what others would do in my situation?

Everything seemed to be going wrong, but yet I felt absolutely right. I wasn't overeating, I was getting plenty of rest, and I had just discovered some amazing correlations in the book my father had given me. I didn't allow the small problems to bother me—I wasn't writing like I had hoped and my thoughts weren't arriving as they had back home, but I felt like I was preparing for something great, that some revelation was at hand.

~ Your Personal Notes ~

12.

I rose just as the sun spread over the baby-blue water. What a view! What a spectacular morning!

Someone flipped a switch. A perfect day was in the offering: a sunny, seventy-four degree, cloudless day.

I took a long walk down the beach; I noticed a man who looked like a native fishing off of the beach. I introduced myself. During our conversation, he told me he loves to cook for tourists; and he pointed to his home just off the beach. He and his wife love their life together and especially enjoy welcoming the travelers to their homeland. He showed me one of the conch shells; that he collected, painted, and sold as a souvenir. While we were speaking, his nephew, who's twelve years old, walked over and introduced himself. We greeted one another with an elaborate handshake as if we'd known each other for years.

We exchanged some pleasantries. When he asked why I was in the Bahamas, I told him I was writing a book on weight loss.

He said, "I don't understand why Americans are so overweight."

He'd watched Americans come to the hotels for many years. "All they do is eat and eat and eat and then lay down." He shook his head. "I just don't understand why they don't go for a walk down the beach or move around after eating."

I told him my goal was to help those people by writing this book. "I think I have the cure," I said.

"When it's written," he asked, "Can you come back and help my mom?" He pointed to her.

I said, "Of course."

"I just want to make sure she is healthy."

"You are a great kid," I said.

I was delighted a twelve-year-old child could identify a problem that afflicts so many while on vacation. Children are intuitive; they, unlike most adults, continue to approach the world with a sense of awe and wonder. Unfortunately, our world tends to strip us of that joyful, intuitive, empathetic nature. What if we could hold on to our childhood grace? We can. The future, surprisingly, does not belong to the children but rather to the adults who mentor and guide our children of tomorrow.

The most significant way we can overcome our country's epidemic of childhood obesity is to lead our children by example, to confirm for them their caring, optimistic attitude is the key to long term health and prevention for weight gain.

Parents hold the key to conquering childhood obesity. Our children love us and look to us for guidance and direction. If we lead by example with healthier lives, healthier thoughts, our children will most likely be healthier and follow our lead. We will have to make real the change in ourselves as adults to change the trend. Those who have children can utilize their love for them to develop a desire to create a healthier model. We can take a stand as mothers, as fathers, and as adults and lead by example. When we become healthy and positive, our children will most likely emulate our behaviors. I have seen this in nearly 100% of mothers I trained; when mom or dad becomes intrigued with health and a positive optimistic attitude, the children eventually become interested, too.

In the majority of households, mothers are the glue and the foundation. They have the passion and the ability to overcome any obstacle, even one as large as the biggest epidemic our country faces. We just simply need the right approach.

Here's an important truth: you are in control of yourself, and your children's society is your home. You have the ability to model for your children the right, truthful way to live and act. Mothers, you can be a great, guiding influence to your children and others around you. Your success depends on you becoming a person who communicates and speaks in a true manner.

When children see their parents eating healthier, being happier, living a happier life, they grow up desiring to walk in the same path. They will want to be like their parents: good souls, genuine people who are living a healthy and happy life. We can't be hypocrites. We can't tell our children to be happy when we are not; we can't tell them to lose weight when we are overweight; we can't model for them a joyful attitude if we have a sour, negative world view.

We love our children; we should love ourselves as much as we love them. The good path we follow will be ready for them, too.

I had my iPod with me, and the boy, Jackson, asked if he could listen. We each used one ear bud. Once the music started, we danced. His uncle laughed at our antics, and Jackson smiled broadly, all his teeth showing. I lent Jackson my iPod for the day. He was grateful and excited. I felt suffused with joy that I could bring such happiness to a young boy.

~ Your Personal Notes ~

13.

I sat on the beach watching the birds and the waves until I decided it was time to sit in the hot tub. Back at the resort, I noticed more vans parked out front; apparently, the tourists had arrived. They were kids, mostly, traveling to the Bahamas for Spring Break. Suddenly, the hotel was busy and full of life.

I walked up some steps and eased into the water where the streams of the jets were pressing into my back. I stared into nothingness. The heat and the mist from the churning water isolated me. I felt as if I were the only one in the hot tub and at the resort. Suddenly, my mind populated with thoughts, thoughts true and real. I pulled myself out of the water and sat on the decking beside the hot tub while my feet remained inside the water. I had to write. The notes poured out of me, naturally and unforced. My patience was paying dividends; the inspiration and the timing converged, and I wrote.

Once I completed my work, I put my notepad aside and slid back into the hot tub. My thoughts wandered off, and I felt again as if I was in another world, alone and undisturbed. Once my mind filled again, I dried off and walked to the beach where I recorded my thoughts for about an hour.

The trip, already delightful, was now also a professional success. I had a notebook full of notes and a recorder full of terrific thoughts—and I still had another day!

I thought I might go out and indulge in some tropical night life, but I decided I might spend my time more peacefully. Something told me to go to bed early so I could wake up early and see the sunrise; perhaps I could collect and record my remaining ideas. I set the alarm clock and went to bed.

I woke before the alarm could sound—and fortunately, too, because I had failed to set the alarm correctly—I could have slept through my final morning!

I packed my essentials and walked until I discovered an area on the beach that was completely secluded. I was about a half a mile away from the resort. I sat in silence and watched the sunrise over the water. The ocean seemed dark until the sun lightened the rising surf. At first, only a small rim of sun appeared, and then with enthusiastic brilliance, the day burst open, and the world radiated goodness. I'd not seen a sunrise so dramatic and startling.

I set up my flip camera and took notes on my thoughts. I didn't force my writing; I sat still, was patient, and wrote when thoughts came to me.

I had a letter that my mother had written to me a few weeks earlier, the only letter I ever received from my mother. I saved her words for a special time; now was the perfect opportunity.

Dear Armando,

Growing up in Italy, I felt as if I were poor because we didn't have any junk food, but the reality was we were not poor after all. Living in Italy, it was easy when it came to eating. We lived a very healthy lifestyle simply because we didn't have access to bad food. I was raised on a large farm with lots of olive trees and luscious fruit trees. We made our own homemade wheat bread, and dinner was a fresh catch of fish, thanks to my father the fisherman. We lived off the land, which had a lot to offer. I didn't know, at the time, just how healthy and lucky we were.

Then one day, many years ago, I woke up in America, a country that we love very much. But one of the first problems that I faced in this new land was the over abundance of junk food that I had never seen before. At first, I did not like American food at all; but I soon got used to it.

And from eating this kind of food, I began to gain weight and not feel good about myself anymore.

After a few years in America, I had my first child, Joe, and then I gained more weight and was not happy about that. Then I had my second child, Patricia, and six years later, unexpectedly, I gave birth to you.

Armando, you were the happiest child. We were always together, and at the age of three you would flex your muscles. It was so cute.

I was always so proud of you and the impact you have had on others. I will never forget what you always say. It's not you but those who hear the truth that are blessed. It is up to individuals to want a better life. You always gave credit to others not yourself. So after many years I finally decided to go to you for help with my weight. Gaining weight over the years began to make me feel depressed when I am actually a very happy person. I never thought that I could workout at my age, but once I started and progressed properly as you would say I never wanted to stop. At the age of 60, I have never felt better in my entire life!

Armando, you inspired me even when I really didn't feel like working out at all. Your smile, your positive attitude, and your overall happiness rubs off on me, and I carry it with me for the rest of the day and every day after that. You are not only my trainer but my beautiful baby boy and mentor! I always gave you what you wanted because you well-deserved anything, and now you were able to give me what I need most. My health and happiness. Health really is wealth!!

I now live by your motto: when you appreciate and have gratitude for your body, your mind, and your health, you can conquer anything. You have taught me the secret to success.

Love,

Mom

My mother's words moved me. I sat for a moment with my eyes closed. I am the one who should thank her—for her kind spirit, for her tenderness, for the millions of genuine moments she sacrificed to raise me. But she was thanking me for restoring her joy, for allowing her to return to the healthy, woman she was in her youth. I had, after all, given back to my mother. I thanked her for being a great mom, and now she was thanking me for guiding her toward truth.

Millions of mothers give to their families as my mother did mine; willingly put their lives on hold to better fulfill the lives of those around them. It is time to give back; I am in the Bahamas and won't stop seeking the answers so every mother's life can be even more blessed! I have a message that is true and real, a message that comes from the depths of my soul, a message that will provide anyone the motivation and the wisdom to change any debilitating habit and achieve weight loss.

While reading my mother's letter two women passed by. I looked directly into my video camera and thought those two women will provide the perfect closure for this trip. There was something special about them. They had pleasant smiles on their faces and greeted me with kind hellos. I sat with my knees pulled up and continued writing. I eventually put the notebook down, turned off the video camera, and started to pack up. I didn't have much time; I had to catch a flight.

I felt suddenly as if time were standing still. As I brushed the sand off my shorts, I saw the two women walking back down the beach toward me. They stopped and walked up to me. One says, "We found these two angel wings in the sand." She handed me two shells; they looked exactly like two wings.

"We were wondering if you could put the wings on and use them to fly home," the woman said. They laughed.

"Oh, I don't know," I said. "You two might have a better chance of that happening. You're the real angels."

They quickly said, "We have to ask you. Do you *Believe* in angels?"

"I've never really thought about it." I smiled. "Interesting you should ask, though. My mother is a spiritual healer."

"I've been studying angels for many years," one of the women said. "We saw you in the hot tub, and I noticed a strong aura around you."

"It was either the Archangel Michael or Gabriel," the other woman said.

"We've never seen anything like it!"

"The glow around you was so powerful, it was spectacular." They seemed to be talking in unison now.

"Really," I said, mystified and delighted. "I don't know much about angels. I'll have to do some research. You've given me quite a compliment."

"We couldn't help but notice you are alone. Why are you here?"

"I'm writing a book."

"We knew it!"

"What gave it away, me writing down notes while I was in the hot tub?" We all laughed.

"No," the taller one spoke now. "We noticed you all by yourself yesterday as if you were the only one on this resort. We couldn't *Believe* how deep in thought you were. It was as if you were in a trance."

"I seem to do that a lot lately."

"Whatever it is you are writing about, we want a copy. What are you writing about?"

I explained *Believe* to them. "I'm dedicating the book to mothers."

The girls eyes began to fill, delighted. "The world definitely needs a book like yours; the mental and spiritual aspect of weight loss. Wow, you are right. This country doesn't need another diet to follow. We need an approach."

They were mothers, one divorced and the other never married. They were on vacation together for the first time. They had decided, jointly, to start living their lives fully. They had felt like victims, unhappy and unmotivated.

"The ultimate message in the book," I offered, "is not just the spiritual and mental aspect of weight loss, but more importantly about being who you were meant to be."

We talked awhile longer about happiness and finding joy and how people cross paths for a reason. I told them I was thankful for their willingness to approach me and share the angel wings with me.

"Our crossing paths were a blessing for me," I said.

"And for us," they said. We hugged and felt like intimate friends, not strangers who had just met fifteen minutes earlier.

I watched them wander away. When they told me they saw an angel around me, the idea didn't shock me. I'm not saying I do or do not *Believe* in angels, but I embraced their kind offering. One could tell by the look on both of their faces that they believed they had seen an Archangel's aura. I knew I had an immediate moment of energy when they saw the aura; perhaps at that moment I was enriched by an angel's presence.

As I walked back to the hotel, I thought about the chain of events that lead me to this precise moment. What if I had become upset when I arrived in my room? What if I complained and argued that I wanted a refund? What If I didn't remain patient the first three days, and what if I changed hotels? If I wasn't an optimist, I probably would have requested a change. If I wasn't patient, when patience was necessary, my life would have 100% changed course for the worse.

I'm immensely grateful for having developed optimism and patience. No fancy room or over-burdened buffet could replace the experiences I had listening to the storm, meeting interesting, inspiring people, and feeling an angelic presence while relaxing in a hot tub.

Just before I turned on to the path taking me to the hotel, I saw Jackson and his uncle. We hugged and shared pleasantries and then said our goodbyes. I let Jackson know he could keep the iPod, but in exchange he had to continue being a great kid. He readily agreed. We all shook hands, and the press of their fingers felt potent—I had made a real connection.

As I walked back to the hotel, I realized that being a good person means we lend a hand when the opportunity strikes—but more than just being kind, why not offer a heart-felt, genuine sympathy. A kind gesture is always valuable—opening a door, smiling, saying hello—but lending our hearts by guiding and giving more hope to others who are in need is priceless. When we guide others who are in despair or in need, they at any moment could become believers in themselves and see their inner passions and gifts; and then with the right positive mindset that we all can have, they will undoubtedly be able to accomplish their dreams and goals that are of truth. You possess the ability to see your inner truth of goodness and health; you have the ability to see, pursue, and make real your dreams. Once you own the reality of your dreams, once you *Believe*, you will succeed!

Our lives can change on small bumps in our daily life—an eye-opening conversation, a shared sandwich, a dance. When one person's life changes for the better, the effect is exponential: the goodness from the single change is paid forward, and others receive the gift of transformation. When one person uses his or her own gifts and talents to help someone else, that other person has the power to help another, and another.

The possibility of change, of individual, communal, and societal change is real. One by one, we will transform into our more resplendent, happier selves, and when we have a culture of joyful, positive individuals, the current world way of thinking will transform, too. Remember, it is not you who need to change; the habits you formed need to change! **When you change for the better, you are becoming the person you are truly meant to be!**

First, we need to make the change real in our minds. Once we *Believe* in truth, the rest follows naturally, and *"the truth shall set you free." John 8:32 NIV*

~ Your Personal Notes ~

14.

My journey home was pleasant, and my life continued with work and writing. One Saturday morning, I decided to play golf, but before I reached the first tee, my phone rang. It was my mother. She told me she had just read the palm of some guy she came across. She informed him about his life, his past experiences, and aspects of his life, and he said to her that she was remarkably accurate. Her gift fascinated him. Turns out, he was a publisher. He offered to be the ghost writer of a memoir of her life, how she came to America from Italy and her special spiritual gift given to her by her grandmother.

I could hear the excitement in her voice. I congratulated and encouraged her. Before we got off the phone, I asked her if she had signed any contracts or if she had any information about the publisher. She gave me his number. I wanted to call him and make sure he was reputable and that he would take good care of my mother. After a great round of golf, I gave the publisher a call.

I called the publisher, and we discussed my mother's book. Because I have been fortunate to work with lawyers as clients, I knew getting the details of the publication process in writing was important. As we talked, the publisher commented about my mother's fascinating gift.

I didn't want to distract him from the topic, but I said, "Not to take away from my mother's story, but I think I have something that you might be interested in." He was game. I told him a small part of my story, and by the end of the conversation, we had plans for him to come to my house that weekend to meet me in person.

When Michael arrived, we greeted one another with hearty handshakes, and from that moment I had full trust in him. I showed him around and encouraged him to feel at home. We sat under the veranda, and I filled him in on the journey thus far and my weight loss theory. I shared with him numerous thoughts about why I was writing a book. I discussed with him why I *Believe* mothers will conquer our childhood and adult obesity epidemic and how I am dedicating the book to mothers. He turned to me and said, "Armando, I truly *Believe* you have a best seller."

I looked him in the eyes and said, "Personally, I have no doubt in my mind." My faith is not egotistical; I am writing *Believe* because the book contains the absolute truth. My theory provides the missing link for those struggling, for those who are overweight and/or obese, and the foundation to one's weight loss and life. He said, "Amen. I *Believe*!"

Michael encouraged me to produce the manuscript and offered to provide an editor. He had a contract to me the next day, and thanks to the phone call by my mother and the patience I demonstrated in allowing the story to unfold naturally, I had a publisher and a vehicle to get my message out.

Michael and I scheduled a second meeting about a month later. The night before Michael was expected to arrive; Michelle and I finalized the manuscript and decided to talk about the book. Michelle and I walked to the veranda. Michelle faced the driveway, and I sat across from her facing the woods on the right side of my property. The breeze was cool; the trees seemed full of life and energy. On the table were three lit candles, notepads, and Michelle's phone to use as a recorder.

While Michelle was getting prepared, I flashed back to all the great moments thus far during the journey. I was inspired. I felt the angelic energy descend on me again. I thought I will never forget this moment. I just felt it. I began speaking, and Michelle turned her phone recorder on. I remember looking at the phone twice to confirm the recorder was on. I had nothing planned to discuss that evening. We had no outline in front of us. I simply began to speak, allowing my subconscious thoughts to rise. Words were flowing more so now than ever. Everything started to seem clear; each word and thought felt crystalline, pure.

There were moments when I spoke so deep from within my soul that Michelle started to cry. I then began to shed a tear. I was more than in touch with what I was saying; I was feeling the words and the thoughts. The words poured out of my soul. I felt my soul speaking nothing but truths; everything left to be said was recorded. I relived moments of my journey, capturing every bit of detail. I elaborated my ideas on how to achieve weight loss and maximize our potential. I completed the book. I felt a moment of perfection. The experience felt unreal, and yet I had just created something very real.

Michelle and I were smiling, beaming with joy, because until that moment, I never understood how I wanted the message to be delivered. I had just finished the overall message of the book, and I had the story on tape. We had completed the first and most important part of the journey: I had a story to tell that could begin a movement.

Our excitement was tangible. Michelle said, "I'll get started typing!"

And I said, "I'll call Michael!'

We had completed one part of our destiny together.

Even though we were scheduled to meet the next day, I called Michael to share with him the revelation Michelle and I had just shared. I was simply too excited to wait.

Michael caught the fever. He was on his way.

I couldn't help myself; something told me to keep going, so I did. Michelle pressed record. We were back in the story. I talked about why mothers are the foundation and the key to conquering our nation's adult and childhood obesity epidemic and how our country's obesity epidemic is a tremendous opportunity in disguise.

Often, we live in what we feel are our comfort zones, pursuing a life that is stagnant and stale, a life some call safe from the unknown. But what do we gain? Very little. The "unknown" is actually our truer selves, the person we were meant to be; what society tells us is the mask. The unknown is what we discover when we *Believe*. Our world within is full of beautiful possibilities and endless joys.

Change, or at least the process of change, comes with uncertainty. Many fear uncertainty in the same way some fear stress—we should avoid stress! But stress makes us strong; when we lift weights, we stress our muscles to become stronger. When we pursue change, we stress our sensibilities, our pessimistic outlook, and our inhibitors that have kept us from living a fully realized life.

We were all born with an essential grace and goodness. And through life, we evolved, made choices, and grew to be the people we are today. If an individual made choices that are further from the truth, those choices lead that person to evolve a life they weren't meant to live. The little choices we make chart the course of life we take. We either choose the path of light and truth or wander off in darkest night. There are truths. Regardless of the religion one follows, certain truths will never change. What will change are the lives of those who seek the truth. Accept the truth, accept the possibility of change, and completely surge into one's true self as the fulfilled, happy, lighter person you were meant to be.

Excellent choices lead to a ripple effect of blessings, and less perfect choices—when truly acknowledged and learned from—are opportunities and can lead one back to the true path with even greater growth and new insight. It's the beauty of not being perfect. We are not perfect. We will make mistakes. We will wander off the hardened path now and then. The key to success, though, is quickly acknowledging when we have strayed and to continue living your life.

We each possess special gifts and talents. A more meaningful life is about seeking and discovering our personal, unique gifts, talents, and abilities. Life is about using them and being the light for others who need guidance and support. Isn't it? Seeking and utilizing our gifts is how individuals and our country evolve. It's what makes this world a better place.

As adults, we need to be the light for our children and others, to lead by example becoming fully empowered individuals. We were not meant to be a population that is over 70% overweight. We as people were not meant to be 20 to 30 to 40 or more pounds overweight. The beauty and passion that mothers possess will grasp onto this truth. Why? Because mothers have the greatest motivating factor to overcome any obstacle their children and our children of America experience. Children desperately need leaders. Children need mothers who are strong, happy, and stress free so they can grow strong-minded and *Believe* in their dreams becoming a reality.

Along with their unique talents and gifts, mothers have a special gift. Mothers are the creators of life! But remember mothers, that you have much more than the complex, wonderful creative force inside you. You have unique passions, talents, and aspirations. Shouldn't we all want to live a better life, to become the light for ourselves and for others? At times we can take for granted our desire for happiness and goodness. The question is not "Do we want happiness?" Of course, we do! The question becomes, 'How do we achieve success: how do we tap into our potential, lose weight, become happier, and in turn share our happiness with our children and others?'

You could list your talents; and if for a second, you say you can't or don't have any, think again! Each of us is gifted in one way or another. But what about those special, powerful talents that you haven't tapped into yet—that you don't know exist within you but most certainly do? The ways we can grow as an individual are endless, and the depths of our power are great. Reaching one's divine destiny is priceless. Ultimately, we should strive first to become the miraculous person God meant us to be, to fully achieve our destiny. Why weight loss and divine destiny? How are the two related? Think about this. There are hundreds of millions in our country who are overweight who are still successful. Are they living in the divine? Fact is enriching our body with natural foods, fruits, vegetables; etc. is scientifically proven to enhance one's mind. We simply function better as human beings. The potential for growth in this country of hundreds of millions and as individuals who are overweight is exponential.

We could ignore our potential; much of our country already does, and consequently, many continue to gain weight, become unhealthy and lethargic, and just go through the motions. Some allow the spark of spirituality to remain dark at their core. But why? Something better is available; why not seize it? If one says it's too hard, change is not easy, they are not recognizing the truth is available to us; the truth is within us, and that change is easy. Imagine a world where our talents are expressed and appreciated, where we are not angry and stressed, where our children see us model health and happiness and grow into their own content, successful lives.

We need to *Believe*—*Believe* first in our own goodness and talent, in our own worth, and second in the potential each of us carries.

And of course, fathers are an essential component of the equation, too. Mothers alone will not revolutionize the world, but their energy and enthusiasm and dedication will be a driving inspiration. I have spent my life watching mothers, talking to them and hearing their stories; I train mothers, and I know how the power of their convictions can light the way for a child. Parents have an inner beauty; both fathers and mothers can become models for their children. Mothers, with their generous, nurturing instincts, will lead the way.

This transformation hasn't happened yet because most haven't heard the truth! Non-believers tend to make excuses. Life is too hectic; I don't have time; it's too hard; I'm too old or too far gone. I am here to tell you that no one is too far gone, and anyone who believes in our innate possibilities and in truth, will prevail.

I wrote a letter to my sister who has traveled to hell and remains. For ten years now she has remained in a world most of us won't ever see although I *Believe* she will beat the odds. I *Believe* she will find this message, and she will hear the truth.

> To my beautiful, brilliant, loving, and amazing, sister,
>
> Patricia,
>
> You have been through a life struggle and let a substance take over you for the past ten years.

You have been through the worst of the worst; you have been through it all, and it's not over yet, and no one is giving up on you.

You can battle your addiction; you are young and have a whole life ahead of you. If you just *Believe* and know that you have the power to do so within you, you will defeat and conquer your battle with drug addiction. Who cares what anyone has to say about anything you have done in your life? You can learn from your mistakes, you can move forward and back on the right path. Just think of the possibilities of what it is that you can achieve and what lies ahead of you. A whole life of success and complete and utter happiness. A family who stands by you and loves you dearly awaits you at home with open arms.

I would hope that one day you are going to read this message I am sending you; but if you don't get the opportunity, I just know and have faith that you are, one day, going to hear this message. One day, you will be blessed with hearing the truth.

But the change begins the moment you *Believe* in a new, better you! I hope you will, eventually, embrace the realization, and then the affirmation, that the change doesn't mean adding an additional burden, but shedding all the burdens that deny growth. A system, a program, a guide to self-actualization to weight loss denies the ultimate truth of you seeking and honoring your mind, your body and your truths. All the knowledge one needs can be sought. All the wisdom you need happens daily, and the best trainer you can ever have is within you every moment along the way. If you *Believe* in yourself and your destiny, if you embrace the truth, then all you have to do is wake up each day and let the beauty of life unfold.

You are the one in control of your own destiny. You are in control of your weight and addiction. Seek your truths. Allow your gifts and talents to shine and become who you were meant to be—not a product of a pessimistic society, not a product of another diet, system, program or Armando, but a product of faith and destiny.

Love,
Armando

~ *Your Personal Notes* ~

15.

While I was talking in to the recorder, I noticed Michelle staring into the sky above us. I smiled. "Michelle, don't worry. Focus."

She returned my look, a bit sheepish. "Armando—look." She pointed heavenward. I was in the middle of a revelation of thought, so I continued talking. After a moment, she couldn't help herself. She pointed above my head. "Armando, you need to look."

"I know, Michelle, I know." I, too, felt something and stopped talking to look.

"There's some kind of mist above you."

I had felt a presence, but my thoughts kept me from looking at and noticing what was around me. I stopped for a moment to fully appreciate the beautiful, peaceful, calming, floating cloud above me. The mist was pure and gentle; I had no doubt it was a spirit of some sort. I felt extremely calm; I could feel the presence of the divine.

Within seconds, the mist formed a line toward me and entered my body. A great force entered my body; I felt like I was about to burst. I was completely paralyzed. I couldn't move my mouth. I tried my hardest to tell Michelle not to worry.

"Oh my God, Armando, what's wrong?" Michelle screamed. She was frantic, crying as if something horrible was happening. I used every ounce of energy I could muster to raise my two fingers and signal her the peace sign to show I was okay. She saw my signal that I was okay and sat back in her chair. I was stuck in a trance.

No mere words can describe the absolute joy I felt. I felt like I was freed from the greatest stresses and anxieties; I felt complete purity as when a baby is born, all the love, all the carefree nature a baby has at birth. I felt an utter peacefulness. The world seemed to slow—no birds, no stars moving, no ticking of a clock. Tears of happiness began to flow. I was ecstatic. The grace of a divine force had descended upon me, entered me, and made me its own.

Even though I was paralyzed, I knew the force was benevolent and that, ultimately, the energy would revitalize me. My book was complete. My message was delivered to me and ready to be delivered to others.

I couldn't wait to share the message with others as I know in my heart of hearts the truth had been given to me and that I am assigned to trumpet the message. A divine force had inspired me, and I just spoke the secret to weight loss and a happier, fuller life.

Within minutes, I was able to move. I said to Michelle, "Did you see that? Wow!"

Her lips were quivering, "Yes. Armando. God filled you." She put her hand on my arm, "While you were speaking about the beauty of mothers and the possibilities to come, how this country can conquer obesity through mothers, a mist started to form and became stronger and stronger." She paused to catch her breath. "I watched it form. Each word you spoke, the mist grew. Two different mists formed above you. Only one entered as the other disappeared."

She looked into my eyes and confirmed what I already felt, "Armando, a spirit joined with you so you would know you were speaking truth." She hesitated. "I almost cannot *Believe* what I just saw." I pointed above her head. As she spoke, a mist had formed above her. She jumped out of her chair and ran behind me. The mist was glowing; the shape shifted, but the outline was in the form of an angel—beautiful and real. The formation of the angel floated for a moment and then quickly dissolved into the air.

I felt astonished and peaceful. Every care disappeared. The world was good and full of happiness. All my goals were attainable. Obstacles were removed: I saw only possibility.

I noticed we were still recording. I asked Michelle to shut it off and to begin transcription immediately. We had recorded the words of a divine force working through me as an agent for change, an agent to inform the world about how to take control of our lives and our destinies, about how to lose weight and become happier during the process.

We changed our location to the kitchen and sat in amazement.

I said to Michelle, "I met two ladies in the Bahamas, Maureen and Kathy, and they thought an aura emanated from the Archangel Gabriel or Michael." I paused. A mystery was being solved. "My publishers name is Michael, and he literally came out of nowhere. Your name is Michelle. Perhaps the Archangel Michael visited us." We were willing to live with the mystery. A divine force visited and entered me; giving the energy a name was not as important as knowing a generous spirit had guided me toward my revelation.

That night, I brushed my teeth with tears of joy streaming down my face. The world had opened up for me; my book would share the truth, and I could realize my dreams. I could share with others the power to realize their dreams.

~ Your Personal Notes ~

16.

The next morning, I woke at 5:30am full of excitement and a sense of inner peace. I felt as if the book had already sold millions and helped millions and I had already reached my goal. I was eager to meet my publisher and present him the manuscript.

I had a full schedule of clients. Michael would arrive at 3:30pm. After meeting with my appointments, I sprinted to my office to read the pages Michelle had prepared. As I entered, I found Michelle sitting on the couch near my desk; she looked as if someone had passed away.

She said, "Armando, it's gone."

"What do you mean it's gone? What's gone?"

"It was recording the whole time, and now it's all gone. Gone! Vanished! It is like we never recorded anything."

"What do you mean all gone?" I heard her, but I couldn't quite *Believe* her.

"It's gone. I don't know. I called the manufacturer of the phone, I called the phone provider and I explained to them what had happened. They couldn't understand why. It's just gone!" Michelle repeated "It's gone," but I didn't want to hear her.

Perhaps I would wake up and laugh at my nightmare.

"I—" words failed me. I had seen the light indicating the phone was recording. I checked multiple times to confirm we were recording. What could have happened?

"We still have two of the recordings, the two from inside the house. We have somehow lost the two recordings from outside."

Michelle sat silently. I knew she felt the same pain—pain as if someone had ripped our hearts out and shown them to us.

My life's work, my divine mission, the realization of my true being: gone in a moment, disappeared as if it never existed. My words floated into space and were claimed by darkness.

I cannot express the pain that ran through my body, a pain deeper than the realization that the audio recording of my thoughts did not exist. My words were gone forever. I felt I could not bring them back. How many times will we receive divine inspiration? I didn't *Believe* I could repeat them.

My euphoria from the previous night evaporated. Numbness crept across my shoulders and arms. I felt the weight of the world descending upon me.

Michelle and I stared into each others' eyes, hoping we could find solace. At just that moment, the doorbell rang. Michael had arrived. I greeted him soberly, brought him into the living room, and sat him down.

He smiled but seemed confused. He had expected excitement.

I explained the dire situation to him. I explained the project was crippled, that the recordings had been lost and that the book could not be written.

Michael listened patiently, and then he said, "Armando, you always tell me there has to be a reason, that you can see the positive in unfortunate events. Don't lose your faith now. You have to *Believe*."

I looked at him.

"It's not for you to figure out, but to *Believe*."

Michelle said, "Michael, what do you mean?"

"Perhaps there is more to the story. Something else is going to come out of this, something good. These kind of unfortunate turn of events plague all of us. The best authors feel they are on to something big, and then, boom, they lose the idea or they change their mind." He paused. "Almost always, something better comes along. I've also heard that energies from spirits distract the frequency of recorders especially those that are not battery operated. It seems as if the two of you proved this to be true."

I considered his argument. I felt, instinctively, that what he said had merit, but losing the recording had sucked the life out me. The truth of what I had recorded was tangible, and I felt it had been stolen from me. The best, most accurate, most moving part of my journey was now missing.

Michael said, "You know, Armando, you obviously have it in you to do this." He smiled.

We talked for a while. He assured both me and Michelle that nothing was really lost, that all I needed was to start again. "Perhaps," he said, "A fresh perspective will bring even greater knowledge."

~ Your Personal Notes ~

17.

My depression did not lift quickly. I couldn't seem to let go of the agony that losing my recordings created. After three days of mourning, I felt I had a choice. I was seriously contemplating not finishing the book. I could take the easy way out and not continue.

Then I gave myself a pep-talk, a serious lecture on the inappropriateness of giving up. Giving up seems like the easy way but feeling defeated and giving in to despair always makes life more difficult. If we give up on finding our deeper purpose, we aren't living the life we were born to live. If one feels it's too hard to eat healthy, for example, giving up and eating junk food might seem easier, but thirty or more pounds later when it's difficult to walk, when one can't climb stairs because he or she gets out of breath, when their doctor tells them diabetes is a risk factor, suddenly they realize they have chosen the wrong path and that which seemed easier had significant, negative consequences.

Ultimately, not pursuing our dreams, not completing our goals will only make life harder. Suddenly, we become listless, depressed, and pessimistic, and then everything we do is colored by our failure. That's the truth. Transplanting one tree at a time, pursuing our goals optimistically and with dedication, will yield practical results and, more importantly, provide habits that will allow for success with all our endeavors. You can walk fast on the wrong path, but only darkness is at the end of that path; if you choose to walk steadily on the right path, you will walk into light.

I know I have a gift I need to share with others. My writing is not about making money; I decided to write because there are hundreds of millions who *Believe* and will hear the truth. I am one of the most positive, optimistic people I know, but the loss of my recordings pushed me into a negative space. The negativity grabbed hold of me, and I quickly neglected the beauty of the spirit's visitation.

A spirit had entered my body and emboldened my soul!

And I'm crying about a few lost hours of me talking? I'm going to give up on the last 10 years of my life, on the wisdom I've gained and need to share?

My faith returned. Michael's words echoed. Something good will arise out of what, at first, seems like misfortune.

At times we all get knocked down, depressed, and angry. Even the most optimistic person can be infected by the virus of pessimistic thinking. We can resist; we can combat the disease of a negative world view with our optimism, with our belief in ourselves and our destiny.

I allowed the virus to infect me for three days. I was miserable; I achieved very little. I temporarily lived a dull, angry life where I couldn't appreciate the beauty of the world around me.

Losing the recordings was not a form of punishment or an act of cruelty. A divine plan, a plan whose shape I couldn't see yet, was forming around me. I trusted in the plan. I trusted that something greater than what I felt I had lost would emerge. I believed the world was working for the good and that I could achieve my goals if I stayed positive and continued to *Believe*!

I felt inspired again. My work would continue, and because I understood the truth to my revelation, this message would help millions of people and I felt even more inspired to carry on. There are people who *Believe*! They are those who hear the truth!

~ Your Personal Notes ~

18.

Angels appear when deep truth is expressed and carried out. Often, those truths are expressed in letters.

Later that evening, I noticed a letter on my counter. I wasn't sure who it could be from other than Michael or Michelle, so I took the letter and went up to my room.

Armando,

At this moment, I lay here crying uncontrollably like the time my mother held me in her arms when I was in despair and in need of the warmth and love that every child so desperately seeks from her mother at a time of sorrow. But this time those tears were tears of refreshment and rejoicing. A calming cry, a cry that was cleansing. I had just witnessed and experienced a kind of miracle. The beauty of the light above you will last in my mind and soul forever!

Every moment, every word, every time you spoke with such passion and deep appreciation for mothers and what they can accomplish in this world by digging deep and finding their true passions and gifts was divinely inspired. I never really thought that mothers would be the foundation necessary to conquer our childhood and adult obesity epidemic, but you made it clear and brought absolute truth to how it could happen. The impact that I have seen you have had on your clients and the impact that it has made on each and every single one of their children gives truth to your theory that mothers are the catalyst for changing this world.

Like you said, just think of the impact one mother living the truth can have on another and then their children! Whether it's one, two, four, or ten, the possibilities of what this world can become are endless.

I lay here continuing to think how you said, from one mother to the next our world will conquer more than just obesity; we can live in a world of complete peace as each one of us builds our character and becomes who we are intended to be. Just as I did.

The message you shared with me tonight goes deeper than mothers just feeling like a mom. You said that the one thing you have heard time and time again over the past ten years of you training mothers is that they feel as if they have lost part of their identity after having children. The feeling of emptiness comes with not becoming who we were meant to be, and if we dig deep and find who we truly are, that emptiness will be vanquished, and we will feel whole again.

Tonight through your words, expressions and emotions, you showed me how you truly feel; there is nothing more precious and valuable than a mother and the love that she gives. Her feelings for her children are what most can't even put into words, but her actions speak more than words. Our mothers in this world are leaders; their children are their motivating factor; and in turn, they will follow in their mother's footsteps. When mothers lead by example, learn from their mistakes and realize that struggles aren't truly struggles, they will propel not only themselves into the future but their children as well.

When we realize that our struggles are really opportunities, and if we go through our obstacles rather than around them and we learn from our mistakes rather than push them aside, we will continue to grow as individuals. We progress rather than regress. If we go off of the true path, we simply get right back on.

There it is again. I lay here, and in my mind I see that mist; that soft, floating, peaceful mist and the peace that it brought to you when it entered your body. At first I was frightened, but after I knew you were okay, I felt at peace. It was breathtaking! I just can't seem to get it out of my head. Every moment that you spoke so deeply, so passionately, the angelic mist appeared.

The time you spoke of how it is possible for us to come out of the economic recession just by one person losing weight and applying the truth to his or her life is remarkable. You are right! The only way you can find that truth of yourself is through believing in the truth of life, of striving for perfection. Striving for perfection is the answer to anyone's success to weight loss and life. As you said, mothers leading by example, demonstrating the truth of weight loss and by being who they truly are, transforms the idea into a movement that is stronger than any infectious disease because this country is in desperate need of just that.

If our obesity epidemic could be cured by a quick fix or pill, not one of us would develop the characteristics needed to grow as an individual. We would never take our life to another level and discover our weaknesses; we could not discover the truth about why we have chosen bad habits and how we can form healthier ones. Our body would lack essential nutrients if we simply took a pill. I am in awe of this approach you have discovered and how it can conquer weight gain, weight loss, and stimulate economic recovery. Sure bailouts might help the economy and diets might help us lose weight temporarily, but the only guaranteed solution requires individuals to grow and evolve and accept truth.

We have an opportunity to use our obesity epidemic and this crisis to touch over 200 million people who are obese or overweight. Each of those 200 million people can achieve a far greater benefit than weight loss. There are qualities that will be discovered about oneself that can be used to grow this country so we can come out of our economic recession. When you first said this tonight, I thought to myself, what a bold statement, but there is such truth behind it all because there is no better way to lose weight other than the individual's way. I just can't get over it. There are 200 million people in this country who can be healed without medicine as a last resort. The healing power is in each and every person who hears and seeks the truth about how it is possible to discover who they truly are, not what they have become because of society. Our obesity epidemic as well as our economic recession can be conquered if only even half of mothers heard this truth and spreads this message simply by leading. From each mother, each family, and each individual to the next, we together can conquer obesity. It's that simple!

Like you said Armando, we live in a great country, and throughout the years, technologically it has grown light years in a matter of minutes. The advances that our country has are amazing. The one thing that could propel us into the future and put us at a level of success that is almost unimaginable, but yet easily achievable is all of us coming together and taking a stand to fight this obesity epidemic. As we all know through the facts, through the truths, human beings who fuel their body with nutritious foods experience many incredible benefits; mentally, physically and spiritually.

The magnitude of the change is enormous. Imagine 200 million people who are overweight enhancing their lives by eating healthier and enriching their bodies with the foods from the earth. By eating healthier our minds become clearer. People instantly feel better as they know they are on their right path, a path that can't be mistaken, a path that's the truth, a path that is real and uniquely special for each and every individual.

I never thought until tonight that adult's unhealthy habits are contributing to childhood obesity. We all want what is best for our children, and as you said, it is up to us as adults to do the best we can, and that's not by just trying but by being. It's up to us as individuals to explore our gifts, our talents and re-discover our identity. By being a nurturer to your children, your family, and everyone around you. There are millions who want to live in a better world and want to raise our children to live in a better world.

We need to grow as individuals. You made it clear that you are not pointing fingers at anybody and you are not saying that anyone is better than anyone else. You firmly *Believe* in your heart that no matter how far off someone is right now, when they look at themselves, they may feel like oh my God this makes sense and I can't *Believe* I let myself get to where I am; it's okay because what they are going to learn about themselves and their life is going to transport them to their divine.

As you said, it doesn't matter how long the

road is to taking the weight off and changing for the better. All that matters is the individual knowing that they are going down the right path. The direction that you are pointing people in is the cure to one's success. The path has been laid out. As we walk the path, we discover our true talents and gifts—we learn as we journey. The path never ends; there is always room for us to progress as an individual and seek the inner depths of our existence. We know we are losing weight for the right reasons--for our children, our family, and our well being. When we *Believe*, we begin understanding how unhealthy it is for one to be overweight, understanding the chances of developing diseases, and how we can decrease stress and anxieties by freeing our body and our mind.

Seek your divine destiny and divine inspirations. So true!

We will and can conquer our difficulties together, and our success depends on us coming together to make an impact and a difference on one another. The people who can start the change, the people who are at the foundation of it all, those who are at the core and the center nucleus of it all, are mothers.

I can't thank you enough for allowing me to experience this journey with you. After what I heard you speak of and what I saw tonight, I wanted you to know the depth of the impact your words and discovery has made on my life. What I saw tonight confirms the truth and beauty of what you have to say. The glorious mist will be a memory I will share with my grandkids some day and one I hope they will share with their children as well. I am truly blessed!!!

—Michelle

~ Your Personal Notes ~

19.

I researched the Archangel Michael on the internet:

According to Michael Brown and Dawn Light/Sacred Circle Hoops website's (found at http://www.creation-science-prophecy.com/michael.htm and www.sacredcirclehoops.com/archangel.htm#mich), that I found on the internet, Archangel means, "Chief of the angels. Michael is one of the two leaders of the angels. His primary functions include ridding the world of fear and toxic energies and assisting with individual's careers and purpose. Michael helps us find our purpose and goals. He can provide us with signs or give us direction regarding our careers and motivate us to move forward by removing fears and negative thinking. Michael boosts our confidence and courage. He is present when we feel threatened or when we need extra faith and confidence or self-esteem to perform a task; he offers emotional support. When communicating our needs to Michael and open ourselves to receive his guidance and protection, we can fulfill our desires and goals."

The other primary angel is the Archangel Gabriel:

According to Dawn Light/Sacred Circle Hoops, DNA Alchemy.com, and Lynx Graywolf website's (found at http://www.sacredcirclehoops.com/archangel.htm#mich, www.dnaalchemy.com/archangelgabriel.html, and http://morningstar.netfirms.com/gabriel.html); that I found while researching on the internet, "Gabriel does the will of God. He is a teacher and a messenger of truth. He has historically provided Leadership. Gabriel can help us fearlessly tap into God's power, and he reassures us that it is safe to contain and exemplify God's power. He is a protector.

"Gabriel appears in the Bible as a messenger on important occasions. The messenger of Spirit, Gabriel brings us good news in abundance! The energy of Gabriel is used to draw many messages of good news that uplift our spirits and help us to feel more fully connected with the universal mind and energy. Gabriel alerts us to be awake and aware, to pay attention to what messages we in turn are giving out to the world and universe each day so that only the best may be sent out to return to us as even more beneficial energies.

"Gabriel works through affirmation. Affirmations inspire us, fill our minds and hearts with hope for a more positive present and future, and support us in turning the great power we all carry within to manifesting the most wonderful life we can imagine."

Angels offer us guidance and protection. We, as individuals, are responsible for leading and directing our own lives. However, we can ask Michael to help us discover our passions and connect them with a fulfilling career that provides for all of our material needs. And Gabriel protects us in our search to affirm our passions and goals."

We are always receiving messages from the Universe; the angels and their great force is all around us, and yet we often walk right past the signs that they designed to answer our questions, to guide us; they provide sign posts that lead the way to our greatest success and fulfillment.

When the Holy Spirit grabs hold of the believer, the Spirit purifies and empowers the soul; the Holy Spirit protects the soul during the spiritual warfare of living in a world that rebels against positive, genuine truth.

May the spirit be with you. **Allow spirits to manifest within!**

While doing research on the internet, according to Robert Longman, Jr. website (found on www.spirithome.com/experien.html), the Holy Spirit means, I came across the following, "When the Holy Spirit inhabits a host, the mechanism is not always clear. Many Christians *Believe* that Baptisms infuses the body, but many others *Believe* the spirit is always alive within us from the moment of conception. For nearly all of us, the spirit is barricaded; we don't recognize or release the genuine, holy spirit that we've locked away in our hearts.

"Christian Pentecost's talk about being 'filled with the Spirit' or having an 'extra portion of the Spirit.' They speak in tongues or are taken over by the Holy Spirit, becoming its conduit. I've heard the assumption of the Holy Spirit described as 'infilling,' 'filling,' or 'fullness,' 'activation' 'enrichment,' 'new openness,' 'awareness,' 'consciousness,' 'awakening,' 'empowerment,' 'recommitment,' and 'reorientation.'

"Catholic charismatic's sometimes use the term "release of the Spirit," suggesting the presence of a greater force further the graces associated with baptism and confirmation. Some Latino Pentecostals speak of *tomada del Espíritu*, which relates the joy of being taken over by God.

"The New Testament, the common experience of believers over the years, and even simple observation testify that the Holy Spirit is not equally present or equally in action at all times and in all people. There are special times when someone with true faith feels the power of angels, of the Holy Spirit, more fully. A calling, a feeling, an intuition: sometimes, this generative force encourages an individual to mature in his or her faith, and sometimes that energy encourages someone to step forward to better serve Christ.

"Mainstream Christians acknowledge the Spirit can come especially at a unique time and place for a particular purpose; in worship services, Holy Communion, and ordinations, they formally call on that same Spirit for precisely such a special presence. Pentecostals know that the Spirit doesn't come only at those formal times, but can do so at any time—whenever it best suits the divine purpose."

No matter our name for the divine presence, no matter the location or formal rites that evoke the spirit, each of us lives in a divine world where the greater forces—whether they are angels, the Universal Mover, the Holy Spirit, Michael or Gabriel—can inhabit our bodies and provide us guidance, repair our confidence, and inspire us to pursue our goals.

I enjoyed such a moment. I felt the presence of a force far greater than I enter my body and shake me to my core. That force saved me and a message to guide and help millions; that force pushed me to continue my journey and to spread the word of self empowerment.

~ Your Personal Notes ~

20.

Once I regained my enthusiasm and positive perspective, I began taking notes and reconstructing my ideas for the book.

Michelle approached me one day and said that Michael was looking for a date to release the book. I didn't want to put a date on anything. Michael wanted to move the process forward; he had practical aspects of publishing to consider.

I said, "You know, something's telling me September 14th." I had a vision of September 14th in my mind. I didn't feel obligated to make my vision a reality, but I would try. I prefer to see a project progress and not measure its success by artificial timelines or scales like in weight loss. My experience as a trainer taught me that gradual progression day in and day out will allow anyone to achieve my goals—not setting dates and no need for weigh-ins.

With weight loss, setting deadlines impedes the day to day progress toward achieving our personal goals and character development. Setting unrealistic goals that are out of one's control is counterproductive. All that matters is the task at hand; we need to continue to learn, grow, and evolve. The rest will come. It always does. Reaching a goal is important and good, but we can't sacrifice the beauty and pleasure we will encounter during the journey.

I will never forget a client who helped me learn this lesson. She had severe struggles with being overweight. She had been training for over four months. She walked in one day with a huge radiant smile. She told me she felt the best she had ever felt, better than she could ever remember. She was fitting into clothes she couldn't remember wearing and compliments were coming to her all weekend. She was ecstatic! She asked if she could weigh herself. I said, why? Who cares? It doesn't make sense to weigh yourself unless you aren't going to get upset and you are just curious. Please keep in mind what you just said. Doesn't that matter most?

She said, "Well, I just want to see where I am." She said, "I just had to."

She was surprised to discover she had not lost as much weight as she thought. She was only down 30 pounds and thought she had lost more. She was distraught. She cried and wanted to quit. She didn't want to move on. All the wonderful emotions she felt, the compliments, and the new habits she formed were in danger of being abandoned.

Gratitude for how one feels and the progress one makes is what is essential, not what the scale says. Weight loss is tricky. The scale may or may not move at certain times during the journey. One will always lose weight, but no one can determine how much, how fast, or how often, certainly not any system or program. Let the pleasure in your progress manifest and be your driving force, not a scale! The weight will come off. Don't focus on the scale; rather, focus on the progression and positive feelings that are energizing you every day.

She learned a valuable lesson; she chose to *Believe* and continued her progress. She lost the weight she hoped to lose and she was happy along the way. She could have been miserable and given up, but she learned from her mistake, remained patient, and had gratitude in each little success that amounted to her reaching her goal. She taught me a valuable lesson.

I decided to plan a four day weekend to complete my book. The trip felt like a great idea but I wasn't sure where I should travel to. I had no strong intuition of what location would be most inspiring. I chose not to choose a location and to see where fate deposited me.

I packed like some women I know: I brought everything! Sometimes, I feel I have developed into thinking like a woman. —I was fully prepared: golf clubs, fishing poles, recorders, video camera, a large variety of clothes, enough for several wardrobe changes—I would be ready for whatever I met. I left my house with a full tank of gas. I drove about a quarter mile and pulled over on a side street and just sat in my car. I thought earlier I might head to the beautiful scenery of Vermont, but suddenly Vermont didn't seem like the best spot.

As I sat in my car, I asked myself, how often do we rush through life? How often do we try to force issues and not trust our feelings and instincts? I'm not sure how many people would have stopped to allow the inspiration to come or just hit the road and forced their trip to happen. In this instance, I didn't have to be in a hurry. I didn't have reservations. I didn't have prior engagements or obligations. A thought arose. **Be still!**

Hmm, where should I go? I sat for about ten minutes and remained still. The day was peaceful. My situation was comical: I had pulled over with a car full of luggage, a book to write, and no place to go. I listened to the rain hit the windshield with a still clear mind, and then inspiration hit me. Litchfield, Connecticut.

Be still to find the answers.

I heard of Litchfield casually. A client told me she found the town peaceful, a place, she said, I need to visit one day.

I searched my texts until I found directions she had sent over a month earlier. I had been looking for a place to go, and she suggested Litchfield. At the time she told me, I didn't feel inspired to travel to Litchfield. My patience and intuition was now paying dividends.

~ Your Personal Notes ~

21.

It was a beautiful day for a drive. Light rain fell from a sky only half full of clouds; the sun peeked through for brief moments. I was enjoying the scenery and the calm feeling that had come upon me. The drive was spectacular. Once again, the sun seemed to guide me. I kept watching down the highway, and once again said to myself like I had in Newport, "That's the direction that I'm supposed to be going."

There was not a car on the road, and every radio station I turned to played my favorite songs. I heard six or seven great songs in a row, and I thought, somebody likes me up there!

When I left the main road and headed toward the town, the scenery overwhelmed me. Trees, mountains, beautiful birds, and the sun peeking through the clouds lit the world. I continued to drive a few more miles until I realized I had missed my turn—I had been enjoying my surroundings. As I searched for a spot to turn around, I noticed a beautiful, white church on my right hand side and up ahead a quaint, little Inn that had to have been 100 years old. I took a mental note and turned around; I knew what turn I had to take now.

I drove with an excited sense of anticipation—I didn't know what to expect when I arrived. As I turned onto a little road surrounded by a canopy of trees and tall grass, a gigantic eagle swooped down along the front of my windshield. The bird's wingspan literally stretched from one side of the car to the other. I stopped the car and watched as the eagle followed the road and then rose above the trees. The power of his presence made my heart stop. I had never been so close to such a magnificent bird.

A series of rich and complicated emotions overwhelmed me. A moment of revelation was at hand, and I knew the truth would be revealed to me.

Other than the eagle and nature, I was alone. I stood still in complete peace and serenity. The light rain subsided, and a beautiful mist rose. I felt a drizzle, but I wanted to walk.

I saw what looked like an entrance to a hiking trail. Once out of the line of trees, I could see I was on the outskirts of a large tract of property, probably thirty acres or more. The path led me to a beautiful grotto. The circular area glowed with hundreds of candles. Not all were lit, but the twenty illuminating the darkness radiated tremendous light.

I could feel the presence of God in that light.

I lit a few more candles and placed money in a donation box. I had discovered the Stations of the Cross. After I said a prayer of gratitude and thanks, I headed over to a posted sign that would explain the Stations of the Cross.

I had never been much of a religious follower. The religious iconography was a mystery, but I could feel energy trembling all around me. Each station led to another station, about fifty or a hundred feet apart. I seemed to grow lighter as I climbed.

At the top of the hill, the drizzly rain stopped and the sun emerged from behind the clouds. I stood at a station. As the warmth of the sun hit me, I glanced ahead to an opening in the trees. My knees buckled, my heart stopped. At the top of the hill, a statue of Jesus bearing the burden of His cross towered above me. I stopped to touch Jesus' hand at the previous station. I closed my eyes and imagined the pain he suffered for us. He bore excruciating pain so we could be free from sin. He died so we could live the lives we were meant to live. He died to certify and empower our faith, to help us *Believe*.

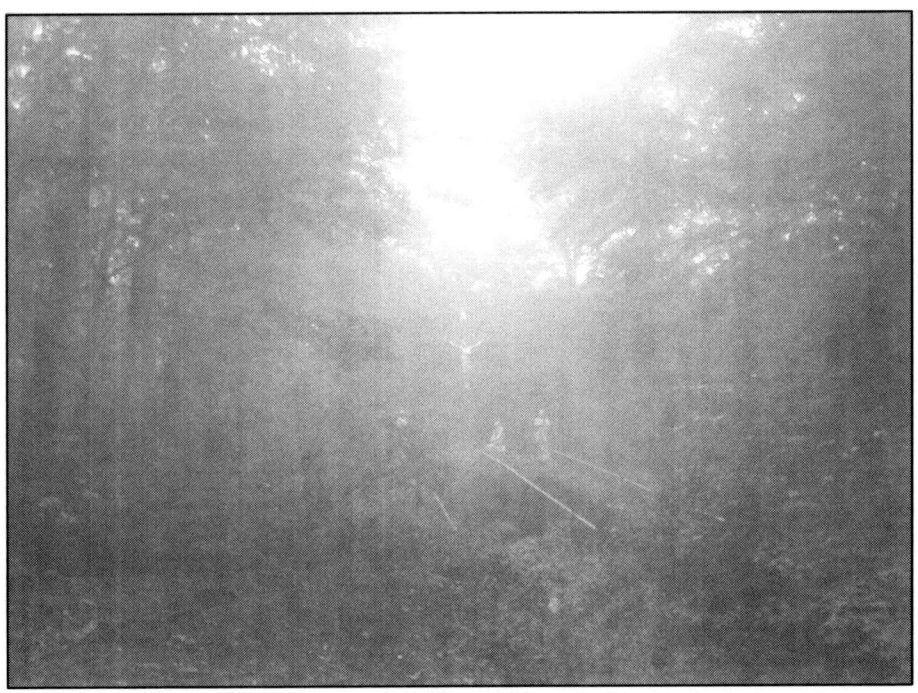

The power of Jesus' sacrifice swept over me. He embraced all the darkness, all the weakness, all the pessimism and angst that could easily crush us so that we could be free to enjoy extraordinary lives. The cross on his shoulders, his burden, was really our own negativity, and he was willing to assume our obstacles and impediments so we could be free.

I felt intensely focused and in-tune to the meaning of Jesus' life. I felt simultaneously his pain and his energy, his kindness, his desire for humanity's success. I felt whole. Suddenly and with amazing certainty, I knew I had discovered the truth, the meaning to my journey. Even through the lingering mist, I could see clearly. God, in whatever form, was the answer.

The truth I always knew but had never fully understood appeared before me, Jesus Christ on the cross over sixty feet tall. The sun fell directly on Him. The air was still, and silence filled the air.

I walked up the flight of stairs toward the magnificent statue and read a plaque placed at the foot of cross: The Twelfth Station, Jesus is Crucified: Feast of the Exaltation of the Cross. September 14th rededicated. My knees buckled and again a feeling that overcame my body was even more powerful than it was throughout this entire journey. The vision of September 14th was real!

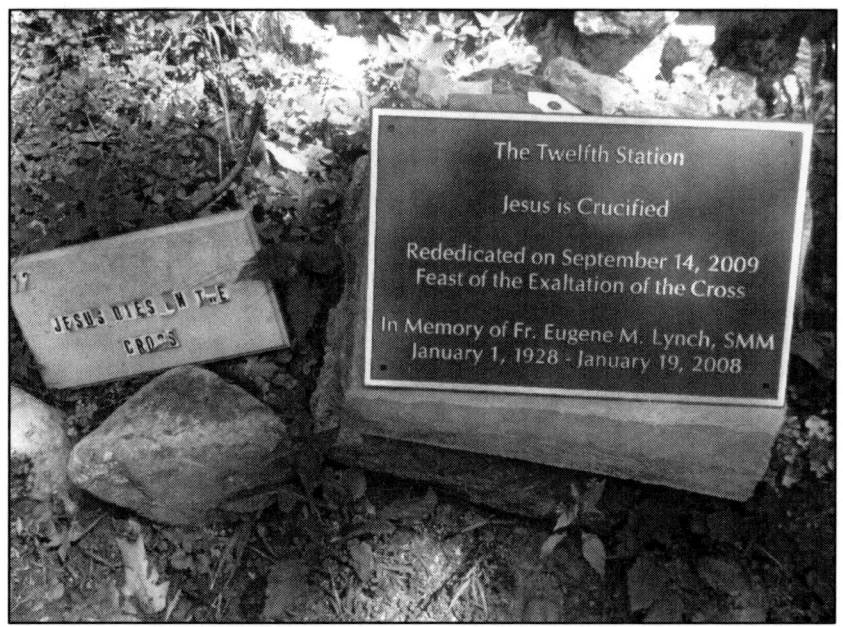

    For most of my adult life, I thought I had a gift—of intuition, of kindness, of understanding. Now I realized I had been walking with God the whole time. When I thought I was trusting my instincts, I was really listening to God. When I was being patient and waiting for a sign, I was really making myself quiet so I could hear the divine speaking from inside me.

> *"Let your patience show itself perfectly in what you do."*
> *James 1:4 NCV*

    I sat in quiet contemplation at the foot of the cross for an hour, allowing the potency of my discovery to take root in my soul. I could now acknowledge God and his primacy in my life. I had found the truth, a glorious truth worth following. My peace, my equanimity, came from God; Jesus would lead me.

"Be still and know that I am God."
Psalm 46:10 NIV

Once I felt that the presence of God had filled me completely, I searched in my backpack and pulled out The Holy Bible my father had presented to me in Newport. Before Newport, The Holy Bible had been an interesting book full of insights, a book unfortunately I rarely opened, but now I held in my hands a revelation of spirit and truth. The book that glowed in my hands felt warm and inviting.

"For it is God who works in you to will
and to act in order to fulfill his good purpose."
Philippians 2:13 NIV

~ Your Personal Notes ~

22.

It's not only about believing in God. If someone asked me the question, do you *Believe* in God, my answer was always yes, but in ten years, I never did anything knowingly to seek God. I got lucky. I decided at a young age to enhance all areas of my life.

"And Jesus grew in wisdom and stature,
and in favor with God and men."
Luke 3:52 NIV

There are 2 billion Christians in this world who *Believe* in God. How many of them are allowing God to guide them? How many are utilizing and seeking their deepest gifts and talents? How many are living in utter peace? How many are overweight and are seeking for answers?

"Through faith we understand that the worlds were framed by the word of God, so that things which are seen were not made of things which do appear.
On the other hand, when you live in faith, you are fearless. One of the best things about having a spiritually-based approach to life is that it allows you to live in a state of peace and confidence instead of the stress and frenzy that characterized the way the world lives. Instead of always being vulnerable to some form of fear or worry, you live in the confidence that there is a Plan, that you are part of it, and that your true needs are being taken care of."
Hebrews 11:3 NIV

So what is the truth to weight loss and living your divine?
The word of God.
The Truth.

"In Christ are hid all the treasures of wisdom and knowledge."
Corinthians 2:3 NIV

Jesus said, "If you hold to my teaching, you are really my disciples. Then you will know the truth, and the truth shall set you free."
John 8:32 NIV

Truly imagine what you are about to read.

Imagine living a life where on a daily basis for the rest of your life you were excited to go to bed because you couldn't wait to wake up, where throughout your day you felt passion, excitement, and peace. Where worries and anxieties were nonexistent, stresses were short lived, obstacles were always overcome and looked at as opportunities, and troubles and setbacks that came your way by making poor choices were learned from.

Would you want to live that life? Stupid question. Of course!

With a renewed mind, it can happen!

"Do not conform any longer to the pattern of this world, but be transformed by the renewing of your mind."
Romans 12:2 NIV

The truth is, accomplishing the transformation of your mind and the revolution of your spirit is not difficult. From the first day you *Believe* the change will be easy, you will feel as if you have reached your goal. All it takes is acknowledging who you have become, seeking the truth, hearing the truth, and living the truth while knowing that one will never be perfect but always striving for perfection.

Every day is going to be a new adventure. Every obstacle will be an opportunity; any trouble or setback that you will go through can be learned from and appreciated. The change doesn't require much. Apply your new state of mind toward your approach with weight loss. Whether you need to lose 20 pounds or 200 pounds, from the moment you *Believe* in the truth you can lose the weight, you have already begun to accomplish your goal.

Your way is the only way!

Your Beliefs. Your Truths. Your Signs. Your God.

"I can do all this through him who gives me strength."
Philippians 4:13 NIV

~ Your Personal Notes ~

23.

The Holy Grail is a symbol of the spiritual wholeness that leads a person to union with the divine and any desired ambition or goal. The Holy Grail culminates a sacred quest and offers each of us a substantial vision of the rewards and benefits our dedication will produce (www.thefreedictionary.com; and appears on back cover).

You can start the process of transformation simply by being who you are. We are not talking about a program that asks you to change yourself to fit into some specific guidelines; the opposite is true: you determine the journey. We are each unique, and each of our journeys will be different. Trust your choices and allow the process to unfold, steadily, over-time—you are revolutionizing your mindset and the consequences will appear in all parts of your life, including your weight loss.

Only two people are controlling your progress: you and your God. As you make choices, it is up to you to listen to the advice and guidance of your personal trainer and life coach, your God.

It is essential at the beginning of your quest that you be honest with yourself. Think about the formed habits and behaviors that have lead to your weight gain. Ask yourself, in what ways have I contributed to my negative mindset and bad habits? Admit to and acknowledge your weaknesses and strengths.

Those who are overweight are not meant to eat the amount and type of food they eat. We can learn to control our bad habits, even if they are old and ingrained habits—even if we think we love the life we have now! Knowing that poor choices are leading toward ill health and disease, we can form new, better habits even if it feels like bad habits are the truth. The only truth is the wisdom that leads to your health.

If you *Believe* in God, let him work miracles in your life. Each day, allow yourself to live life and enjoy the richness of your experiences. Be aware to the greatness all around you. Have gratitude far greater than having thanks. Feel the divinity of your potential in your soul—the foods that are grown from this earth, the scenery around us, the lives of those special to us.

"Examine yourselves to see whether you are in the faith; test yourselves. Do you not realize that Christ Jesus is in you - unless, of course, you fail the test? And I trust that you will discover that we have not failed the test. Now we pray to God that you will not do anything wrong-not that people will see that we have stood the test but that you will do what is right even though we may seem to have failed. For we cannot do anything against the truth, but only for the truth. We are glad whenever we are weak but you are strong; and our prayer is for your perfection."
2 Corinthians 13:5-9 NIV

Our lives are divinely orchestrated. The scriptures talk about how God has already written all of our days. He promised His plans for us are for good and not wicked. God will use everything we go through to move us toward our divine purpose. Regardless if we go left when we should have gone right. We need to stay on the true path, and when we go off the path, we simply learn from our experiences and get back on. Such right thinking will always lead you to success. Transforming your life is that simple! No guilt, no worry, no rules. Live and acknowledge.

When you know your life is divinely orchestrated, you *Believe* that things are not happening to you—they are happening for you whether they seem good or bad. You may stray and make what seem like unfortunate choices, but even those are opportunities. God can make any poor choice into an opportunity to learn from. All one needs to do is to acknowledge the truth to ones mistakes. Everyone who believes and is overweight can acknowledge their truths and the importance of eating healthily as well as the importance of maintaining a healthy weight.

Those who are 20, 30 or 40 or more pounds overweight are most likely overeating and overindulging in foods that contribute to their weight, foods that are human-made and processed. As human beings, we were not meant to eat processed food as regularly as we eat natural foods, but over 70% of our country is habituated to eating processed food.

Perhaps you have unhealthy eating habits—and perhaps you love junk food and think that a candy bar is a reward, is a pleasure you can't live without. For some of us, junk food is a hobby! I argue eating junk food is a habit—and a habit one can break. I've never seen a potato chip field or a cupcake tree. The natural world has innumerable treats for us—strawberries, cashews, kiwis, whole grains, fresh water, cantaloupe, blueberries…. I could, of course, go on and on. What I can assure you is that the less you indulge in sweets, foods that are high in fat, foods that aren't natural, the less you will crave them. Make healthy foods one of your hobbies and allow the unhealthy foods to disappear from your desires; you desire them now because you are used to them. Once you develop an optimistic mindset and a belief in the value of healthy foods, and eat them consistently, they will become just as much of a desirable choice.

We make choices; we are responsible and accountable for our behaviors: we grab the food with our hands and put it in our mouths. If you are one who has created a habit of overeating, overindulging, or regularly choosing foods that aren't conducive to health, rest assured: the moment you acknowledge your truth, your weaknesses, and your mistakes, God will use your confession as an incredible opportunity for growth far greater than any diet, program, or system could ever accomplish. Your past eating sins will be a blessing, and you will be enlightened the moment you *Believe* in this truth. Not because I say so but because you *Believe*!

> *"Who forbid marriage and require abstinence from foods that God created to be received with thanksgiving by those who believe and know the truth. For everything created by God is good, and nothing is to be rejected if it is received with thanksgiving, for it is made holy by the word of God and prayer."*
> *1 Timothy 4:3-5 ESV*

If you decide you need support and some form of structure, trust your instincts; there are many useful plans and products that can help with weight loss. I encourage you, though, to trust in God and allow the process to develop. I encourage you to be aware and receptive. With weight loss programs, you may lose weight, but if you don't gain knowledge and wisdom— you will most definitely regain the weight or struggle the rest of your life. A new attitude that is grateful, optimistic and a mind that seeks knowledge and wisdom is far more powerful than every product in the entire weight loss industry put together.

> *"For the LORD gives wisdom; from His mouth come knowledge and understanding. He stores up sound wisdom for the upright; He is a shield to those who walk in integrity,*
>
> *Guarding the paths of justice, and He preserves the way of His godly ones. Then you will discern righteousness and justice and equity and every good course. For wisdom will enter your heart, and knowledge will be pleasant to your soul;*
>
> *Discretion will guard you, understanding will watch over you, To deliver you from the way of evil, from the man who speaks perverse things; From those who leave the paths of uprightness, to walk in the ways of darkness."*
>
> *Proverbs 2:6-13 NAS*

With *Believe*, guilt vanishes. If you feel guilty, don't, because you shouldn't—not because I said so, but because God said so. If you desire to overcome any poor decisions or choices you might have made in your life, God absolves you of guilt: your past struggles are opportunities for you to learn from and grow from and not hide from or forget. We can't dwell on our past, but we should learn from it. Being thoughtful and aware of one's mistakes, but also willing to let go and move forward, is crucial to anyone's success in weight loss and in life.

The millions of us who *Believe* can alter the way we think, the way we act, the way we move through the world—and the list of benefits are endless. In our world, where technology has taken a central position, we have an abundance of choices between wondrous and incredible innovations, although many are desperately struggling with our sense of humanity. Those who *Believe* feel the change—you most likely sense the world is losing its core goodness. You feel it in the air. You feel it all around you. We can begin to reconnect, to locate and embrace a better way of enjoying the multiple and endless goodness in our world. The transformation begins when we accept the truth, acknowledge and determine to change our negative ways, and seek the truth.

"Do you not know that in a race all the runners run, but only one receives the prize? So run that you may obtain it. Every athlete exercises self-control in all things. They do it to receive a perishable wreath, but we are imperishable. So I do not run aimlessly; I do not box as one beating the air. But I discipline my body and keep it under control, lest after preaching to others I myself should be disqualified."
1 Corinthians 9:24-27 ESV

Your new journey will be filled to over-abundance with the knowledge you gain by seeking truths, with the wisdom you acquire by applying knowledge, and the experiences you enjoy by developing a mindset that is much needed in life and in this world. When mistakes are made, view them as opportunities for growth and learn. Where you are lacking in knowledge, gain the knowledge. Use that knowledge, apply it to your life and gain the wisdom that is far greater than any gold.

"How much better to get wisdom than gold,
to get insight rather than silver!

The highway of the upright avoids evil;
those who guard their ways preserve their lives.

Pride goes before destruction,
a haughty spirit before a fall.

*Better to be lowly in spirit along with the oppressed
than to share plunder with the proud.*

*Whoever gives heed to instruction prospers,
and blessed is the one who trusts in the LORD."
Proverbs 16:16-20 NIV*

When you create for yourself a new mindset of true optimism, of gratitude and appreciation of your body, your mind, your soul and your health, your life will flourish.

We believers can unite and restore the way our country and our world was meant to be. We can strive for perfection in our lives and change for the better; we are not changing who we are; we are becoming who we were meant to be.

*"I'm eager to encourage you in your faith, but I also want to be encouraged by yours."
Romans 1:12 NLV*

The gratitude you will feel toward your new body, your mind, and your spirit will become overwhelming. You will see the signs and you will feel God's presence.

What seems complex, and perhaps even impossible, will suddenly seem simple and clear. The one, evident answer to your questions about weight loss and your one true destiny is to: trust in God.

*"Don't you know you are God's temple and God's spirit lives in you."
1 Corinthians 3:16 NIV*

Having deep gratitude for all that is around us and for all that comes our way, developing patience, developing persistence, having an optimistic and positive attitude, developing a heightened awareness to all that's around you and all that comes your way, changing how you think and why you do what you do, being diligent and persistent, and believing are all qualities that life fulfilling and extremely easy; not difficult and empty!

Luckily, I fell into a belief of seeking truths and a way of forming positive habits. God was my guide—even thought I didn't realize God's presence at first. I took a leap of faith when I believed I had a gift. A gift of truth about how to achieve weight loss. Each person who believes in this truth will accomplish weight loss 100% of the time and begin to live in the divine.

If I hadn't believed from the moment of opening Debbie's letter in Texas, not one word would have been put on paper. If I had taken a shortcut or if I wasn't patient, I would have stopped in Newport when I read those Bible verses for the first time. If I had taken a shortcut, I would not have been led to the amazing signs and on the incredible journey I experienced. All the feelings, the lessons learned, the growth that came out of my journey is far greater than the material rewards of writing a best seller because now I have wisdom. I have learned lessons about how to live a successful, rewarding life. I have not caught a fish; I have learned to fish—and you can, too.

"Now faith is confidence in what we hope for and assurance about what we do not see. This is what the ancients were commended for."
Hebrews 11:1-2 NIV

If I hadn't been optimistic and looked for the positives in each of my setbacks, troubles, or obstacles, I would never have reached success—I would have stopped long before the spirits visited and blessed me. If I didn't have deep gratitude for all life's greatness and the secret power in each of us, I doubt I would be the person delivering this message to you. Life is not about struggling, worrying, having anxiety, and being uncomfortable in our bodies. Life is about enjoying yourself and being happy and helping one another. We can live abundantly, and God's plan will unfold in time for each of us!

> *"It is not for you to know the times or dates the Father has set by his own authority."*
> *Acts 1:7 NIV*

> *"Let us not become weary in doing good, for at the proper time we will reap a harvest if we do not give up."*
> *Galatians 6:9 NIV*

When I was in Newport, I basically knew the truth to weight loss; my vision on the shore was quite potent. I came home that day and opened the Bible, and by chance I turned to a page that spoke directly to me and to my vision on The Cliff. At that moment of surprise and delight, I could have continued looking through the Bible and linked my thoughts to the Bible's truths, but I chose to continue my journey and accumulate more wisdom and experience so my truth would be wholly my own. Perhaps picking up the Bible that afternoon was a sign from God to end the journey, but in the moment I felt it was confirmation to continue on. I'm grateful I continued; I needed the journey and its experiences to solidify my faith. I would have missed the cross in the sky, the white rabbit, the hummingbird, the white squirrel, the angel, and the gorgeous eagle welcoming me to see Jesus Christ on the cross.

I could have finished the book earlier perhaps, but for whatever reason, ending this part of my journey didn't feel right until the moment that Jesus Christ was right in front of me. The date I chose of September 14th was a vision. On that day, everything crystallized. You will have your moment, too, if you haven't already! There are millions who already had their moment even before picking up this book. If you are one who has and has been in search for the answer to your weight loss, God bless you.

You are on the way to your success. I did not learn my truths from the Bible; I learned my truths from the journey and then found they were echoed in the Bible. If I had tried to fit my life to the Bible's truths, I may have reached the same conclusion, but many of the truths might not have felt as real to me. I am grateful for the journey, and you will be grateful for yours—certainly, there is no singular way to reach the truth, but earning our truths sure feels good.

> *"Your word is the lamp to my feet*
> *And the light to my path."*
> *Psalm 119:105 NIV*

We all have choices, and we all can make the best choices; we can and strive not to give up—ever. If you make the best choices you can, by always progressing and never giving up, you will reach your goal. No quick fixes, though some goals take a year, some ten, some a few months. Patience and knowing you are on the right track is the key. Approach your goals honestly and directly; if your eyes are open to your strengths and weaknesses, when you begin to pursue your dreams, you will already feel as if you are at your goal. If you need to lose 20, 30, or more pounds and this message touched you, you are blessed with hearing the truth. That's the power of believing.

> *"Because you have seen me, you have believed;*
> *Blessed are those who have not seen and yet have believed."*
> *John 20:29 NIV*

Potentially, I could have achieved basically the same end result, but if I had taken a shortcut, my connection to God would not be as strong. What I learned in my journey over the past year has enriched my life far more beautifully than any shortcut and any amount of money ever could. My experience transcends the easy fix, the quick answer, the sure understanding—my soul is deeper and my faith stronger. Being a spiritual person is not about being on your knees praying every day; it's not about having to go to church. Of course, prayer and church are great, but the truly spiritual person makes a daily connection to gratitude and happiness, a daily thanks for your body, your mind and your soul.

"Therefore if you have any encouragement from being united with Christ, if any comfort from his love, if any common sharing in the Spirit, if any tenderness and compassion, then make my joy complete by being like-minded, having the same love, being one in spirit and of one mind.
Do nothing out of selfish ambition or vain conceit. Rather, in humility value others above yourselves."
Philippians 2:1-3 NIV

We can form true gratitude for God's presence and guidance, true gratitude for everything that exists around us of truth and of value to our human body, mind, and soul. We need the journey. If I stopped in Newport—which would have been like taking a diet pill or following a program —I might have thought I would have succeeded; but a year later, I would have still been searching. And those who follow a program will be most likely tipping the scales once again and missing the miracles one the journey toward their truths. There is much more to learn; the journey brings wisdom; wisdom brings continuous and perpetual success and not just momentary pleasure.

To truly learn and gain wisdom, we must focus not only on *what* we do but also on *why* we do. We can learn to trust the process and to be intentional as we progress—conscious of our choices and their repercussions so we can gain wisdom. Sometimes, the wisdom we gain through the process of achieving our goal is more valuable than the end goal. Of course, we want to be successful, but more importantly, we want to know how to be successful and why we have been successful so we can repeat the experience for all our choices and decisions. You can achieve one goal or you can achieve one goal and learn through the process how to be successful in the pursuit of all your goals.

The similar truth applies to weight loss. Unless you are a body builder or fitness competitor, you have no real reason to follow a specific diet, system, or program. You can have success with a program, but the weight loss most likely will be temporary; if, however, you're attentive to your choices and learn from your experiences—if you allow the journey to give you wisdom—you will not have to struggle repetitively with programs because your wisdom and subconscious will guide you to consistently good choices that have consistently good results.

Once we acknowledge our weakness, we can form new, healthier habits—progressively, over-time. Your choices become habits, and your habits become who you are—the easy and natural you! You will begin to think about and make healthy choices without thinking. Your conscious awareness will evolve in to subconscious thoughts. But first, you need to be attentive and aware of your choices; over time, they become habitual. You are not conscious of walking or brushing your teeth, but you had to learn to do both; they are now ingrained habits that you simply *do*. As you develop a conscious awareness you become more aware to miracles happening around you.

"I will show wonders in the heaven above and signs on the earth below."
Acts 2:19 NIV

"Teacher, we want to see a sign from you."
Matthew 12:38 NIV

We all have an unlimited possibility of growth, and growing is natural and simple. Pride, ignorance, or apathy can hinder our growth, and each of these is a habit of mind one can eliminate. Once one accepts and internalizes a more positive, optimistic outlook, then the negative forces controlling our choices disappear.

"Whoever slanders his neighbor in secret, him will I put to silence;
Whoever has haughty eyes and a proud heart, him will I not tolerate."
Psalm 101:5 NIV

"For everything in the world – the lust of the flesh, the lust of the eyes,
And the pride of life – comes not from the Father but from the world."
1 John 2:16 NIV

So what is it exactly that you need to be aware of that is going to help you succeed in weight loss? What truths do you need to focus on? All of them and there is no specific order. Allow God to guide you. Let God be your daily trainer. Be receptive to all the truths while showing preference for the ones that have most meaning to you, that seem like important guides or messages for you. You are on your own journey—not someone else's. You don't need me to tell you what to *Believe* or what to focus on—you already know, and during your journey, you will become more certain about what is most important to your success.

You are choosing to become healthier because you want to be enriched by the word of God, but what comes out of your renewed dedication is far greater than weight loss. You will become who you were meant to be.

Learn to be patient. Learn to sit still in the world. Learn to be receptive to signs and the wisdom of others around you. All of these skills make life easier not harder. As you develop each of these skills, you will lose weight, but you will also enjoy the process of becoming healthier because a deeper purpose, a larger belief in the person you will become, motivates you. Losing weight is one benefit of gaining these new skills, but many more advantages will accumulate—and suddenly, you're whole life, and the life of those around you, will be more amazing.

"Finally, brothers and sisters, whatever is true, whatever is noble, whatever is right, whatever is pure, whatever is lovely, whatever is admirable—if anything is excellent or praiseworthy—think about such things. ⁹ Whatever you have learned or received or heard from me, or seen in me—put it into practice. And the God of peace will be with you."
Philippians 4:8-9 NIV

Think about all of the words in the Bible that have a positive force: Awareness. Wisdom. Knowledge. *Believe*. Patience. Appreciation. Progression. Truth. Optimism. Preparation. Gratitude. Foundation. Renew. Accept. Choices. Acknowledge. Diligence. Passion. Moderation. Perseverance. Endurance. Humbleness. Accountable. Discipline. Ponder. Dedication. Seek. Vision. Unity. Strength. Purpose. Search. Timing. Repent. Temple. Thinking. And the list goes on.

From the list, can you acknowledge which words represent your strengths? And which ones represent your weaknesses?

If you *Believe* in God, you *Believe* that God is your father and that God is your creator. God created you to live a life full of abundance. God wants you to live life every day, fully and with passion and with excitement and gratitude by simply progressing in whatever you are seeking to accomplish. The truth is simple, but sometimes we are unable to acknowledge our weaknesses or admit that our habits of pessimism are contradicting God's desire for us to live happily. We might hide weaknesses from ourselves or from others, but one can never hide from God. Thankfully, God will always forgive us; our guilt for past poor choices will disappear once we acknowledge our failings, learn from them, and begin moving in a more positive direction.

You don't have to be perfect. You don't need to worry every day if you're making the right choice. If you make a wrong choice, just simply acknowledge your error. Eating unhealthy on a daily basis is one way of harming one's own body. Acknowledge how you are hurting yourself and develop new habits. Only you know the truth.

God is everywhere. He's not just in church, and you don't have to just go to church to find him. At any moment of the day, at any point of your life, God is available to you. God is your on-call, 24-hour ready personal trainer, your guide; to tap into God's power, all you have to do is acknowledge, be aware, and progress: develop patience, dedication, and persistence. Mirror the positive words of God.

"May the Lord direct your hearts into God's love and Christ's perseverance."
2 Thessalonians 3-5 NIV

"Then I acknowledge my sin to you and did not cover up my iniquity. I said, 'I will confess my transgressions to the LORD' – and you forgave the guilt of my sin."
Psalm 32:5 NIV

Think about all of the words in the Bible that have a negative force: Shortcuts. Worry. Temptations. Discourage. Anger. Pessimistic. Disbelief. Anxiety. Dishonesty. Boasting. Uneasiness. Disbelief. Feeling worthless. Gluttony. Troubles. Lack of faith. Overwhelmed. Proud. And the list goes on.

Do any of these resemble traits you have developed? If so, these words inhibit our growth. Which attitudes do you want to change, what new habits do you want to form?

We can renew our minds, seek the truth, gain knowledge, and acquire wisdom. Embark on your own journey, and God will guide you to the answers!

"Wisdom is supreme; therefore get wisdom.
Though it cost all you have, get understanding."
Proverbs 4:7 NIV

> *"For the LORD gives wisdom;*
> *from his mouth come knowledge and understanding.*
> *He holds success in store for the upright,*
> *he is a shield to those whose walk is blameless,*
> *for he guards the course of the just*
> *and protects the way of his faithful ones.*
>
> *Then you will understand what is right and just*
> *and fair—every good path.*
> *For wisdom will enter your heart,*
> *and knowledge will be pleasant to your soul.*
> *Discretion will protect you,*
> *and understanding will guard you.*
>
> *Wisdom will save you from the ways of wicked men,*
> *from men whose words are perverse."*
>
> Proverbs 2:6-12 NIV

How many times have you said to yourself, "I'll start my diet on Monday" or "I'll start improving my health and living better on January first" or "I'll start better habits when I get back from vacation?" Perhaps you've said no to treats because "I'm on a diet" or "I wish I could eat that but I can't—today's not my cheat day."

The list of awkward things we have to say is endless: I can't eat that lemon bar today, but maybe tomorrow! I really would like to eat that piece of cake, but I need to save my points! I weigh in tomorrow, so no gravy tonight! No carbohydrates for me! Boy, this sucks!

Unless God has spoken to you and asked you to set a schedule, a weight goal, or collect numbers and points toward health, you are wasting your time playing these diet games. Most weight loss programs ask you to sacrifice and, as a consequence, can deny you the experience of gaining wisdom and living a good, happy life. If one wants that piece of cake, and when they are told you can't have it, they tend to feel defeated. They will most likely feel the negative pull of old habits.

Imagine, though, eating that piece of cake because you want it and have made other changes to your diet that are leading toward a healthy lifestyle. You have formed patterns of eating vegetables and fruits and other healthy foods, and that piece of cake is not going to stop your progress. In fact, you may not want that piece of cake after all—you'll want an apple or an orange or a mango instead. Weight loss isn't about denying yourself what you want; weight loss is about habituating yourself to eating, and therefore wanting foods that are healthy. Some feel that a piece of cake is delicious, but where does having a slice everyday leave that person? Unhealthy, overweight, and craving more. When one frees themselves from everyday indulgences, they begin to free themselves of the need to indulge. We don't lose goodness by eating right; we gain health. We do lose the desire for unhealthy foods and negative habits; the longer you practice good behaviors, the easier and more enjoyable engaging in those healthy habits become!

The renewal of your body begins with a renewal of your mind. We need to reorient ourselves, to turn away from negative thoughts and habits and turn toward positive ones. With the power of your mind it's simple with daily conscious awareness. The reward; your renewed mind and subconscious thoughts take over. You'll begin to think without thinking.

> *"In your relationships with one another,*
> *have the same mindset as Christ Jesus."*
> *Philippians 2:5 NIV*

Our society has taught us unhealthy habits. Fast food and processed sugar surround us, and we are taught to indulge and enjoy them—in fact, we are taught they are the path to happiness and we shouldn't deprive ourselves! But we know now that fast food and junk food are not healthy, affect our mood in negative ways, pack on the pounds, and contribute to numerous long term and serious health problems, including diabetes, hyper tension, heart attacks, joint paint, muscle fatigue, and strokes. Moderation!

> *"Accept instruction from his mouth*
> *and lay up his words in your heart."*
> Job 22:22 NIV

> *"Show yourself in all respects to be a model of good works,*
> *and in your teaching show integrity, dignity."*
> Titus 2:7 ESV

Seek a deeper desire to eat healthy, an appreciation for enjoying earth's bounty. You may not currently have that desire and appreciation; culture and society have strong influences on us. Our orientation toward fast food and junk food is a dangerous habit, but our culture tells us that all these quick and easy and tasty foods are healthy and will make us happy. They will ruin our health and contribute to our unhappiness.

You can change your view, though. You can form new and better habits. And, best news of all, the change won't require points and frozen meals or weighing in on a scale every day! You don't have to change your habits over night. Any drastic, sudden changes will be counterproductive. Your willpower will diminish if you simply deny yourself the foods you have always enjoyed.

Instead, re-acclimate yourself to the wonders and joys of healthy eating slowly and steadily—with God's help and on God's timing. Through your belief, you will develop a stronger, sturdier character that will easily overcome our society's negative messages.

God will always respond to someone who is seeking to better his or her life. God wants to empower you to see and realize the possibilities within you, to help you establish and maintain true and useful change. The Bible contains many amazing truths, and each one of those truths is applicable to your weight loss: you have knowledge and wisdom within you, you have opportunities and joys surrounding you, you have the diligence and optimism to make real your true self, and you can locate and embrace the patience and guidance that God offers you.

All you have to do is *Believe*—in yourself and in divine guidance and support. All the points of my journey had led me to this one, supreme truth—we are surrounded by goodness, by a spirit that will infuse us with health and power if we are patient, if we are still and receptive, and if we work toward a gradual shift in our thinking. For all of you who decided to read *Believe* and apply what you are reading to your life, you are blessed! Remember, when you adopt new habits for the better, it isn't change. It's merely you becoming who you were meant to be. Go live the life you were meant to live!

"Blessed rather are those who hear the word of God and obey it."
Luke 11:28 NIV

"Ask and it will be given to you, seek and you will find; knock and the door will be opened to you. For everyone who asks receives; he who seeks finds; and to him who knocks, the door will be opened."
Matthew 7:7-8 NIV

Restore your body to what it once was or where it should be: healthy and nurtured, our bodies are truly our temples, and once we treat them with respect and honor their needs, we can truly connect with a brighter world.

"It is sown a natural body; it is raised a spiritual body. If there is a natural body, there is also a spiritual body."
1 Corinthians 15:44 NIV

If I were to give you in a small, simple packet all the words I spoke on The Cliff in Newport, in the car, all those nights waking at 3am, in the Bahamas, or on the night I was blessed by a higher power in my backyard, I would be cheating you out of a necessary journey. I had to experience my obstacles, setbacks, successes, choices, thoughts, and signs during my journey to gain wisdom, and it is a must to your weight loss journey to be attentive to your trials and successes, too.

Your journey will be exciting and different—we are each unique! The journey is not solely about losing weight; the journey is about seeing the world differently and seeing your weight loss as part of a holistic vision of your place in the world. Once you are content, you will move toward weight loss and over-all improved health. The truth is cyclical: the more you improve your health, the more you will be happy; the happier you are, the more you will feel and become healthy.

I'm sure many of you possess the same traits I developed—you are resilient, caring, curious, and eager to live well; however, you might view the world a little differently, a little less optimistically, and changing your view can make all the difference. The transition from negative habits to positive habits most likely will be easily understood and easily implemented in your life. You simply have to begin! One small step will lead to larger steps; soon, you'll be running!

If you *Believe* in the truth and you *Believe* that you have a greater purpose in life than where you currently are today, when you apply these character traits that are essential to weight loss and keeping weight off, you are striving to live and be the person that God, your creator, put you on earth to be. You can enhance your body, your mind, and your soul. A deeper, more profound spiritual connection will make your journey beautiful and enjoyable. You will achieve your goals because obstacles will be opportunities and even problems are really only moments to prove your power and to deepen your trust that God is guiding you.

> *"Guide me in your truth and teach me,*
> *for you are God my Savior,*
> *and my hope is in you all day long."*
> *Psalm 25:5 NIV*

~ Your Personal Notes ~

24.

What would I do if I were you, and where should you begin?

Live your life as you were before reading *Believe*.

And while you are living your life and enjoying each experience, supplement your life by choosing each day to embrace and seek knowledge about everything you choose to eat. Become wise about how you feel and, especially, about your motivations for your actions. Honestly acknowledge to your God your weaknesses and remain open to receive His guidance.

Become informed about what you eat and drink and understand the benefits or the damage you are doing to your body; everything we consume can do good or harm. Over time, whether it be a week or two or however long you need, you will start developing a deeper understanding of your diet and what you might alter to be healthier.

"Pride brings a person low, but the lowly in spirit gain honor."
Proverbs 29:23 NIV

Learn about protein, the types of carbohydrates, the types of fat, fiber, vitamins and minerals, and antioxidants. Become knowledgeable about food and nutrition, and you will begin to internalize the information that is valuable. Educating yourself is key to transforming your habits because the information will seep into your subconscious and become part of your motivation. When you go to select a meal or a snack, that information will be available to you, and you will make better choices. **It is a must to become educated about nutrition.** The process of learning is important; read a little bit every day. You don't have to alter your schedules and grocery shopping routines and the dinners you prepare every night all at once; the change will be gradual. As you absorb a little information each day—about the nutritional value of fruits and vegetables, about the dangers of processed sugar, about how lean meats are good for the heart—you will naturally adapt your eating patterns and choices to fit a more healthy regimen. Your conscious and subconscious will become linked, and the negative habits that drove your eating choices previously will simply disappear, replaced by educated, positive choices.

> *"A gentle answer turns away wrath, but a harsh word stirs up anger. The tongue of the wise commends knowledge, but the mouth of the fool gushes folly."*
> Proverbs 15:2 NIV

Show gratitude in all areas of your life and especially develop gratitude for the foods God has blessed us with on this earth to replenish our bodies and our minds—foods that are rich with antioxidants, minerals, vitamins, healthy carbohydrates, and good fats. These natural, healthy foods assist with growth and renewal of our mind. Developing deep gratitude is essential! Gratitude will overcome ones feelings of deprivation. Instead of "I can't have a cup of ice cream," know that you can because you are not on a diet and food doesn't control you. Instead, appreciate what you put in your body.

> *"Let the message of Christ dwell among you richly as you teach and admonish one another with all wisdom through psalms, hymns, and songs from the Spirit, singing to God with gratitude from your hearts."*
> Colossians 3:16 NIV

After time, the habits of eating unhealthily will be replaced by the habits of eating healthy. What might have seemed in the beginning a chore (changing the way you value certain foods) will become a pleasure. Eventually you will look forward to eating healthy foods; your desire to eat good foods will develop because they will be appealing and desirable in the same way unhealthy foods seem desirable and appetizing now. If you don't have appreciation for food, for healthy food, for food that God put on this earth, once you gain knowledge on a daily basis to the nutritional values of what is in foods you eat, you will begin to develop a deeper appreciation! Allow God to speak to you! God is talking if we are listening.   Learn what is in fruits, vegetables, meats, whole grains, and nuts. Begin incorporating healthy foods into your diet. With education and slow assimilation of healthy foods, you will transform your eating habits and, by extension, your body. You are gaining healthy habits and losing unhealthy habits. You are not losing the opportunity to eat fried foods; you are gaining the appreciation of a juicy, delicious piece of fruit!

"It is good to praise the LORD
and make music to your name, O Most High,
proclaiming your love in the morning
and your faithfulness at night."
Psalm 92:1-2 NIV

    Gain wisdom as you live your life and introduce these delicious, healthy foods in your life by acknowledging how amazing you feel, how much better your brain and body begins to function, how shiny and rich your skin, hair, eyes, and nails look, and how much more energy you have —simply because you are eating these types of foods. Processed, high fat, sugary foods provide almost no nutritional value, and they certainly don't give your body the necessary vitamins and minerals to flourish. Pay attention when you drink a soda or eat a candy bar and notice how you feel sluggish for two hours once the ten minute sugar rush subsides. With nearly all healthier options, you get a steady, pure, and consistent release of energy, and all good, wholesome foods provide a similar mood enhancement daily and long term. Processed foods create mood swings that most always end in the valley of negative feelings, but healthy foods allow you to climb the mountains of joy!

> *"For attaining wisdom and discipline; for understanding words of insight; for acquiring a disciplined and prudent life, doing what is right and just and fair; for giving prudence to the simple, knowledge and discretion to the young - let the wise listen and add their learning, and let the discerning get guidance."*
>
> Proverbs 1:1-6 NIV

As you gain wisdom, you will become smarter about yourself and your own needs and desires. We all have weaknesses; we all give in to temptations. What are your weaknesses? Once you answer that question honestly, you can begin to compensate for them. You can discover the answers for how to overcome the habits and choices that so far have limited you. You are unique. Ask your own questions and seek your unique answers. You will have your own struggles, but by slowly and steadily educating yourself about what the rich, abundant, natural world has to offer you, you will overcome your liabilities and mature into the person and body you want to be—a person with energy and beauty who is pursuing your passions and sharing your unique gifts.

Once you have acknowledged your shortcomings and worked steadily to overcome the temporary obstacles, the weight will fall off, and you will achieve the natural weight you were meant to be. Don't ever give up! Persevere!

> *"Because he himself suffered when he was tempted,*
> *He is able to help those who are being tempted."*
> Hebrews 2:18 NIV

Perhaps you eat out of loneliness or boredom. Perhaps your parents told you to "clean your plate!" when you were young, and now at a restaurant you feel compelled to eat the entire enormous portion served to you. We all have specific, often psychological or historical, reasons for making the specific food choices we make. Perhaps exercise is too hard or you don't have enough time. Most people don't exercise enough or don't eat the best foods because they have formed bad habits that they justify and rationalize. It's simple to gain weight when we don't acknowledge the root error in our way of thinking about exercise and food choices. We should just be honest with ourselves and work slowly and a little at a time, to form new habits, new ways of thinking that are positive and affirming.

> *"Get wisdom and get understanding; do not forget wisdom, and she will protect you; love her and she will watch over you. Wisdom is supreme; therefore, get wisdom."*
> *Proverbs 4:5-7 NIV*

Please don't be discouraged if you fail or have a setback in any endeavor. You truly can let go of depression that arises from a bad day. Minimize your frustration and forgive yourself. Move on quickly from what might seem like mistakes and setbacks because they are, after all, successes and opportunities for growth and gaining great wisdom!

~ Your Personal Notes ~

25.

When I was in Newport and I began to thumb through the Bible, this is what I stopped on –

"By wisdom a house is built, and through understanding it is established. Through knowledge its rooms are filled with rare and beautiful treasures. A wise man has great power, and a man of knowledge increases strength. For waging war you need guidance, and for victory many advisers."
Proverbs 24:3:6 NIV

There I was reading the Bible for the first time in my life. The Bible confirmed for me the sentiments I had felt on The Cliff —that if we are unwilling to see our errors, and gain wisdom from examining them, then we are doomed to failure and continue to struggle.

Those who accomplish their true potential —in weight loss and in life—are energetic, healthy, and, above all else, curious: they want to learn about everything that affects them, including their mistakes. They understand that knowledge is the key to power, and power is the key to success. By becoming educated about themselves, by honestly assessing their own strengths and weaknesses and then working toward improving their weak areas, they move steadily toward success.

Each of my successful friends and clients searched for knowledge; they gathered information, made sense of it, gained wisdom, and then applied what they had learned to their life. They embraced the possibility of learning from their mistakes and changing their mindset to allow for improvement.

"Blessed is the man who finds wisdom, the man who gains understanding."
Proverbs 3:13 NIV

The majority who struggle with weight loss or in life tend to lack a desire to gain wisdom and knowledge to overcome the obstacles they feel prevent their success. Many people want to be told what to do—it seems easier than educating ourselves and making our own decisions. Unfortunately, many of us get the wrong message. We tend to listen to the advertisers or others who are not educated and who are delivering a false message. We tend to trust them to tell us the truth when really they are only forwarding ignorance or trying to make a buck. Think about it.

We need to take back control of our own lives. We may not even realize or understand that our choices stem from someone else telling us what to do; we never really examined why we like fast food so much, but perhaps the reason we like a greasy hamburger is because our friends like them or the commercials are appealing or because we think it's easier to grab fast food than to pack a lunch. Once we examine the reasons for our choices, we begin the process of taking control. We can think rationally and critically about what we want to eat, how much we want to exercise, and why, and then we can make decisions for ourselves.

Some people seem to be lucky—they can stay in shape and look great with what seems like very little effort. The truth is, though, they have the knowledge, and they know what certain foods they should eat or when they should work out. Over time, staying in shape is actually easy. The majority of us who struggle with weight loss simply lack the knowledge and the mind set for capturing the experience of how to take the best care of our bodies—we aren't ignorant, but we haven't taken the journey to educate ourselves yet. When we gain the knowledge and adjust our outlook about eating and exercise, we can begin to control our own lives and make choices that are healthy and that will lead to increased energy and positive feelings.

Here's a game plan for success with weight loss: learn about the scientific elements of food, educate yourself about your own motivations and choices, and develop in yourself a positive mindset about eating and exercising—and food will never control you again. You will control your food and exercises choices. Those who simply don't want to take control and take responsibility for their choices are destined to fail. Statistics prove this to be true. If you want to take control of your life and get off the merry-go-round of diets then it's a must for you to take responsibility with genuine optimism, gain knowledge, and seek wisdom.

Let's say you binge on junk food or overeat late at night; ask yourself, what is the true reason for why you have these unhealthy habits? Maybe you cite stress—work is always pushing you for more. Now that you have identified stress as the culprit, ask yourself if there is something you can do to eliminate or reduce that stress. Eating will not solve the problem; in fact, eating unhealthily to solve your stress issue will only contribute to your stress—you'll add weight, you'll feel worse about yourself, and your hypertension will increase and then you'll be stressed about those things! Binge eating provides only a momentary satisfaction. Do you eat because you are bored? After you are done eating, are you still bored?

"See to it that no one takes you captive by philosophy and empty deceit, according to human tradition, according to the elemental spirits of the world, and not according to Christ."
Colossians 2:8 NIV

Unhealthy eating is a band-aid for a much larger wound. You will still be bored. You will still feel stressed. Almost always, an underlying issue contributes to over-eating—we are using food to solve some other problem. Seek out those problems. Separate them from eating. Find other solutions to those problems and reserve eating for the purpose of healthy, nutritious, enjoyable replenishment of your body. Try to go for a walk, meditate, and allow your new positive outlook to guide you— the junk food this country has accumulated won't make you feel better. The world is full of treasures, all waiting for you to envision and embrace!

"By faith we understand that the universe was formed at God's command, so that what is seen was not made out of what was visible." Hebrews 11:3 NIV

~ Your Personal Notes ~

26.

Before I sought out the truths to my life and gained wisdom from experiences, I never knew life could ever be so invigorating and peaceful at the same time.

For almost ten years now, God has been reaching out to me through many diverse animals, people, feelings, emotions, and experiences. If I ignored them or chose to rationalize them, I wouldn't have made it far on my journey. Take the time to notice the miracles happening daily. Be still. Remain receptive and aware—the good or the obstacles—and don't miss God's guidance along your journey. All of our experiences have meaning; whether they are signs or not, a pattern exists that provides meaning and guidance. Become sensitive to the spiritual world and the messages it is sending us, and one way to become sensitive is to embrace any obstacle as an opportunity to evolve and make your dream become a reality. Allow your journey to be compelling, invigorating, and peaceful. Be open to the miracles in your life.

So Jesus said to him, "Unless you see signs and wonders you will not believe." John 4:48 NIV

"In your majesty live forth victoriously in the cause of truth, humility and justice; let your right hand achieve awesome deeds." Psalm 45:4 NIV

"But it is more necessary for you that I remain in your body. Convinces of this, I know that I will remain, and I will continue with all of you for your progress and joy in the faith, so that through my being with you again your joy in Christ Jesus will overflow on account of me.

Paul had a purpose for living when he served the Philippians and others. We also need a purpose for living that goes beyond providing for our own physical needs. Whom can you serve or help? What is your purpose of living?" Philippians 2:24-26 NIV

We all have had a cold or possibly the flu or an injury, broken bones, torn ligaments. Of course, illness or injury is unfortunate, but it shouldn't take these incidents to remind us of how lucky we are to be healthy, to have true gratitude for our bodies being healthy. Unfortunately, those who are overweight gain weight gradually, over time, and may not be aware of how the weight gain is making them feel. Sluggishness, joint pain, and depression might sneak up on us and feel "normal." If you are 20 or more pounds overweight, think about what you are carrying around all day. The extra weight is excess body, and the stress of carrying that extra weight is significant on joints, internal organs, and our cardiac system.

Try this: fill a five gallon bucket with water--that weighs approximately forty pounds and carry the bucket around with you. Most likely, you wouldn't last more than two minutes. But if you're overweight, you have no choice—you must carry that weight with you, and the burden is enormous. Imagine releasing that forty pound bucket—how light and easy your life would seem! Imagine having the flu but not being aware that you were ill and waking up one morning healthy—you could breathe easier, your vision would be clearer, your chest wouldn't hurt, and your head and sinuses would be focused and crisp. Losing a few extra pounds will be a revelation; you'll feel as if you've shed burdens that have kept you chained and depressed.

"Where there is no vision, the people perish...."
Proverbs 29:18 KJV

"Now faith is the substance of things hoped for, the evidence of things not seen."
Hebrews 11:1 NIV

You need to live your own life. No one diet or plan will fit everyone. Your wisdom will come to you differently than my wisdom came to me; if you're patient, if you learn from your mistakes and make yourself receptive to the wisdom around you, if you accept the process and work toward changing the negative habits that have kept you overweight, you will succeed.

Let's say I was once addicted to foods high in sugar. If I ignored how I felt after I over-indulged in foods high in sugar (jumpy, unfocused, fatigued), I lost a crucial piece of information necessary for the next time temptation strikes. If I paid attention to *how* I felt (and *why* I ate five slices of pizza, half a bag of chips, a pint of ice cream, fried foods), the next time I might not choose the excessive amount or the unhealthy food because I've gained wisdom and know how eating that processed sugary snack made me feel. Embrace the uncomfortable feelings of overeating and poor food choices. Enjoy how amazing you feel after you eat a little less or make better choices.

You can capture and store in your subconscious thoughts and feelings toward how you feel when you over-eat or make poor food choices so that in the future you develop a desire to make different choices when temptations strike (especially in the beginning when cravings arise). These desires for inappropriate foods are common and understandable. Why? For many of us, certain foods are as addictive as drugs like crack, heroin, and alcohol. Many unhealthy foods are processed, human made substances that become addictive because they are full of sugar, fat, salt, and calories that over stimulate your taste buds and mind. These substances satisfy basic evolutionary needs, but we need only small amounts, and we tend to eat excessive amounts.

"No temptation has taken you except what is common to mankind. And God is faithful; he will not let you be tempted beyond what you can bear. But when you are tempted, he will also provide a way out so that you can endure it."
1 Corinthians 10:13 NIV

Luckily, eating foods from the earth can also become addictive! Why? Because we can't ignore how amazing we feel, how good we look, how clear our thinking is, and how wonderful the whole world seems—our family, our friends, our activities—when our bodies are processing healthy foods. Of course, we can eat cookies once in a while—who really wants to give up birthday cake! You don't have to give up all of our processed foods. We need to shift our focus, though, so that natural, healthy foods dominate our food choices, and then the occasional sweet won't hurt us.

Every day, seek a little more knowledge about what certain terms mean; such as, sugar free, fat free, high fructose corn syrup, added sugar, and no sugar added—learn about what you're putting in your body, what the health benefits or risks are of certain foods. Learn to read labels and look up different foods and terms on the internet. If you have children, what is in the food you're offering them? You should know! They don't have a choice, but we do— so let's choose to make healthy choices and to form habits that ultimately lead to our and our children's health and happiness.

We all enjoy tasty food, but what allows us to eat healthy is deeper than the taste. We need to feel grateful for the nutrients in our foods. When we appreciate the benefits of eating an orange; the orange tastes even sweeter. Regardless if you are skinny, have a high metabolism, or not especially overweight but would like to lose just a little, filling your body with foods from the earth is both beneficial and pleasant. If being overweight made me feel good, I would be overweight because why wouldn't I want to live daily feeling the best that I could. But science and years of anecdotal evidence suggests that being at a healthy weight promotes an endless variety of positive life changing benefits; being overweight encourages an endless variety of chronic health issues and behavioral problems, including depression and a negative self-concept.

God has placed before us a bounty of delicious and healthy food, delights that enhance our body, mind, and spirit. God did not make candy cane fields, fried food forests, or liquid sugar lakes— He made necessities for human growth and enjoyment. You are not depriving yourself of something essential when you eat healthy foods. Cakes, pies, chips or fries are not essential. Water and lean meats, carbohydrates, proteins, nuts, fruits and berries, vegetables and healthy fats are essential. We are not depriving ourselves of delicious treats (unhealthy food and snacks); instead, we are learning to be grateful for the healthy, delicious, satisfying, and helpful foods that will make us stronger, happier, and more fulfilled. Deprivation is ridding yourself of a substance one needs to survive: water, air, healthy food. Are we really deprived if we eat healthy or if we eat junk?

I acknowledged at a young age that I was a jealous person; I acknowledged at a young age that I was selfish; I acknowledged at a young age when I was hurtful toward others; I acknowledged all the binges, all the poor food choices, and all the mistakes I was making. By developing a conscious awareness I taught myself how to learn from my mistakes and how to make myself a better, more generous, more vibrant person. You can make similar confessions—and then free yourself from the guilt. We can acknowledge who we were and not feel guilty about recognizing the truth of our past because we are making progress, we are moving toward a truer, more real, more important us—the us we were always meant to be.

Start your journey your way and keep in mind these truths; assess your strengths and weaknesses and simply lessen the amount of junk and include more nutritious foods. Incorporate some walks and exercise into your daily habits.

"For we are God's workmanship, created in Christ Jesus to do good works, which God prepared in advance for us to do."
Ephesians 2:10 NIV

Try doing this if you don't already: walk as if God is walking right next to you. He already is, but acknowledge His presence. Notice how you begin to act and eat. Give it a try. We can become receptive to the grace and guidance that God offers us. Act apart from those who are sabotaging this country and living under falsehoods. Don't be a victim. Be a successor. Establish the traits that God wants in all of us.

"Jesus said, "If you hold to my teaching, you are really my disciples. Then you will know the truth, and the truth shall set you free."
John 8:31 NIV

These traits are related to weight loss and to you finding out who you truly are, where your true gifts and passions lie. The world is full of people who have ignored their talents and traveled down a different path. And yet, there are millions of stories of people who make discoveries, accomplish amazing feats, and live every day with meaning. **You will be successful because you heard the truth and you acted on it. You deserve all the credit!** No program or diet can be credited with your success—allow your power of belief to strengthen your faith and accomplish your weight loss.

Analyze and assess yourself every day. Pay attention to the moments and experiences of your day. Notice how you are thinking throughout the day. If you are a pessimistic person, ask yourself if your negative world view is benefiting you and your situation. It never does! Start renewing your mind by being aware and blocking negative thoughts or learning why they arise. If there is a reason for your pessimism, tackle the problem until you overcome it. If there isn't a real reason and you're simply being angry or mad or defeated out of habit, block and dismiss the emotion. Re-orient to the positive. Your subconscious will develop its own habit of positive thinking. Being optimistic is a learned behavior that evolves by focusing consciously and daily.

"Though the LORD is supreme, He takes care of those who are humble, but he stays away from the proud."
Psalm 138:6 NCV

Be still, but be proactive. Allow the richness of life to become the core of your consciousness. Develop habits of optimism, and you will become an optimistic person in all situations. Allow God to speak to you.

"But Jesus often withdrew to lonely places and prayed."
Luke 5:16 NIV

So how do you go about making better choices? You simply reverse some of the habits that you have ingrained without thinking about them through a slow, steady process of consciously choosing new habits. You change your way and at your own gradual pace!

Recognizing the transformation your consciousness and your body will undergo is not immediate, but occurs progressively over time, frees you to take the journey at your own pace, naturally. In time, you will evolve healthy habits and a healthy body and mind. You have to trust yourself and the process; in the journey, you will find great peace and happiness. You will lose body fat!

"But if we hope for what we do not see, we wait for it with patience."
Romans 8:25 ESV

Let's say you are someone who doesn't do any cardiovascular exercise, but you want to lose weight and you think adding a little time on the treadmill or walks outside would be useful. Well, they most definitely will! If you do an hour the first day you go to the gym, you'll be exhausted, sore and will dread going again and again and again, and will most likely quit. You will not form a habit; instead, you will most likely convince yourself it's all simply too hard. You need to progress slowly, maybe ten minutes a day every other day, so you can get used to the changes and enjoy the sensation of getting stronger without being sore and feeling beat up.

Let's say you travel ¾ of a mile in ten minutes. The next time you do cardio, you do ten minutes again and either increase the incline, which makes it harder, or try to go a little further. You can make small changes because each day you'll progress naturally and become stronger. And, most importantly, each day you'll feel successful and you'll be building a habit of exercise. Soon, you'll be eager to get on the treadmill because you're getting stronger, feeling better, and know you can do the exercise without hating the experience. In fact, you might start to look forward to and love exercising.

On the tree farm, I could have tried to move as many trees as possible on the first day and then worked like crazy for the next week or so, but I probably would have injured myself, gotten terrific blisters that would have prevented me from doing my work, or just decided it was too difficult. Instead, I habituated myself to moderate work each day—work that accomplished my goals without making me hate the experience. In fact, I looked forward to my daily experience of moving the trees just as you will look forward, in time, to your exercise! In all honesty, I don't *enjoy* working out, but I absolutely love the results of how I feel and look—and, of course, the amazing health benefits. I don't think anyone *enjoys* the physical aspect of brushing his/her teeth, either, but we form the habit because we realize the advantages and feeling. After a while, we wouldn't miss brushing our teeth—the habit sticks, and we look forward to enjoying our bright, white teeth and fresh breath!

> *"Therefore, since we are surrounded by such a great cloud of witnesses, let us throw off everything that hinders and the sin that so easily entangles. And let us run with perseverance the race marked out for us."*
> *Hebrews 12:1 NIV*

Perhaps you want to lose weight "right now!" If you think you are going to get more benefits by exercising furiously, you are wrong. You need to work steadier, not faster; you need to work smarter, not harder. You can learn to be efficient. We all know the story of the tortoise and the hare–slow and steady wins the race while furious and undisciplined always loses. You don't have to work out like a hamster in a wheel. Exercise should be pleasant, not a burden; you aren't depriving yourself of time on the couch—

you are having the opportunity, for which you are grateful, to exercise your magnificent body!

What's true with exercise is also true with dieting. You can't expect to revolutionize your diet overnight. Instead, think in terms of small changes that will add up over time. Incremental progression is useful for weight loss, weight training, and every other aspect of life. Examine your current habits and dedicate yourself to construct new, healthier habits. Stay positive and focused and trust that daily, incremental progress will allow you to reach your goal. A lot of times much sooner than one might think.

> *"So do not throw away your confidence; it will be richly rewarded. You need to persevere so that when you have done the will of God, you will receive what he has promised."*
> *Hebrews 10:35-36 NIV*

Be Persistent.

Dedicate yourself to make at least one small change a day. One small change—like one tree or one ten minute walk on the treadmill—will become multiple changes, and soon you will be happily walking for a longer time period, you will have all the trees moved, and you will have a full life of good habits.

Trust that small changes will add up to larger transformations. Body fat will begin to melt away and your mind will be renewed.

Ask for guidance and be receptive, and you will receive guidance. Seek the truth, and you will find truth.

~ Your Personal Notes ~

27.

God will guide you 100% of the time. He won't ever cancel on you to go on a vacation to the Bahamas to write a book. He won't text or talk on a tape recorder during your training sessions. He won't miss any sessions because he is sick with shingles or because he broke his ankle. He won't cancel because he has food poisoning. He won't take time off to go fishing or to play golf. He won't be unavailable when you need him most. God will always be there for you. God has all your answers!

God is available all the time. He is your ever-attentive personal trainer, to answer your questions, support you, and guide you toward a healthier, happier life.

28.

God led you to *Believe* for a reason.

Our country is in trouble. Perhaps you are struggling daily. The world is full of hucksters, liars, and tellers of false truths. Every day, we are offered gimmicks and programs that simply won't work long term.

Let's hold each others' hands and come together by simply being our unique selves, enriched with truth. Our children need us to see and share the light.

Millions *Believe* in the truth. Millions *Believe* in being happier and healthier, exercising, and living a vital, spiritual life.

Millions of us are grateful for our world, our bodies, and the glorious, bountiful happiness that exists all around us.

Are you one of the millions who hear the truth and are on the right path to a more abundantly, rewarding and successful life?

You need only to make a few small changes, one at a time.

29.

A full human life is balanced.

May the wind be at your back when you most need fresh air.

May the sun shine on your face.

May patience be with you when you most need calm.

May you be persistent, evolving into the you being you,

aware of the signs that come to you.

You are God's blessings, and each and every one of us has gifts within us,

unleash those gifts and unlock your potential. Reach for what your heart and soul desire.

You and your transformation are the first part of a larger evolution.

World peace is possible.

Each believer brings light to the next.

Soon the whole world will be ablaze with truth.

Find your deepest passion.

Conquer your wishes and desires.

Enjoy your journey.

Live your life fully and happily and with the light of love emanating from you!

"And we know that in all things God works for the good of those who love him, who[a] have been called according to his purpose."

Romans 8:28 NIV

30.

Share the renewal of your mind with your kids.

Share the energy of your knowledge and wisdom with all those around you.

Share by simply leading by example and being you!

"For lack of guidance a nation falls, but many advisers make victory sure."
Proverbs 11:14 NIV

31.

So how will mothers conquer obesity and restore our country to greatness?

My journey started with a letter from one mother who changed her life, and I end *Believe* with another letter, this time from a child whose mother believed and became healthy; as a consequence, her daughter saw the light. The revolution begins with mothers, with each one of us becoming the light so we can share our wisdom and insight.

Dear Armando,

You probably don't know why I am writing to you, but the reason is I want you to know how grateful I am. My mom was a little depressed before she saw you, but now she is always so happy. She is excited to work out! She is very healthy and eating healthy (although she is eating a cupcake right now, hah!). Mom is starting to run and has lost so much weight, thanks to you ☺. She is happy with herself, and I just want you to know that she is so bright and positive, and I know you are the reason. You are like my second dad, Armando! I love seeing you because you are always so upbeat, and you make me happy!

A year and a half ago, something tragic happened to me. I went to a school, and people were getting sick. To be more specific, they were getting the stomach bug. One day, I started to feel sick and went home. I did not get sick, but I was scared I would. I was terrified of going back to school. I always had stomach aches, and now I know that they were nervous stomach aches, but I wasn't sure back then. I left that school and was home-schooled until March, and then I went back to my old school. I went for very short days; I was on a medicine. My psychologist decided to up the amount as I got back to school, and then I started to get very depressed.

I hated life, and sometimes I threatened to kill myself. It was pretty bad, and I got kicked out until I got an evaluation from my psychiatrist. I was terrified to go back to school, and my mom started to see you. She was always the one to reassure me, and she would always say, "Yes, I promise you are fine." But I would need to ask constantly. Then she got healthier. I was always terrified of something happening to her, but thanks to you, you gave her motivation to workout, lose weight, eat healthier, and live happier.

You changed her life and it also affected mine. Thank you so much! She used to be a little overweight, not exactly skinny, but not that fat either, a little over average I suppose. She always ate a little unhealthy, but as she saw you, she started to be healthier. She stopped yelling and crying and she started eating properly, and then she got thinner, and soon enough almost all her clothes were baggy on her. She was so happy with the results, and to see her so happy it makes me so happy!

I am very thankful for all you did. You helped my brothers Erik and Zack, and they are becoming healthier, too. Max always seemed to work out, but he hasn't seen you yet, but you working with Erik and Zack got him more motivated. You have such a good effect on our family, and we should all be very thankful. My dad is happy with my mom's health, and I know that he likes you, and my brothers like you as well.

I was always very scared of her dying, but now I am less nervous because she is healthier, the risks are so much lower, and just know that I think you are the coolest guy ever! I mean, who could hate you, Armando? You are so sweet, and you have a great effect on everyone! I am still nervous about getting sick, but seeing my mom happier and healthier makes me ecstatic! You really took the edge off my worries. Thanks again!

And now my mom sees you on Mondays and Wednesdays. That just makes my whole week great! Sunday nights are hard. Well, they are always hard for everyone I have to say, but for me I always worried about school. My school starts at 9:00am, so my mom would have to bring me with her to see you because I hated taking the bus, but being there makes my day great! I love being with Michelle and you, and I love having our handshake. I like it when you rub my head and say hi. You brighten my whole day. That is why I love Mondays and Wednesdays! ☺

Armando, I am repeating this for the 20th time, but THANK YOU SO MUCH! You are a great guy, and you are one of the happiest, nicest people I know! Thank you so much, Armando. I really appreciate all that you have done.

Sincerely,
Rachael :)

One mother's situation improved, a positive outlook changed not only her life, but the lives of her children, not by having to follow rigid rules or by telling but by communicating and leading by example. By living and seeking the truth.

You can be the light of your family. You can be the one who starts the transformation for yourself and then share your wisdom with others.

We can all learn from one another by seeing ones actions. To show how to be positive in negative situations, to have a smile on your face that is genuine. You will spread the message by becoming a better you—the you God meant you to be. Just by being you, you will represent the possibilities of true, generous change.

Let your inner beauty shine. One step at a time, one person at a time, we will transform ourselves and then the world!

"And without faith it is impossible to please God, because anyone who comes to him must believe that he exists and that he rewards those who earnestly seek him."

Hebrews 11:6 NIV

32.

The next letter is a true testament of developing a strong foundation by not following a program.

Dear Armando,

As I look over the last 15 months since I wrote the letter that you read in Dallas, I am amazed at the changes in my life. Your mantra "strive for perfection" finally makes sense to me. When we first met, I was content to strive for mediocrity. Unable to see that I was capable of achieving so much more than that, I found myself on so many occasions just doing what was necessary to get through the day. If that meant reaching for junk food when I was stressed or a cocktail when I was bored, I never in those moments understood how I was depriving myself of great things.

The thing that amazes me the most is that my life or the activities of my life haven't changed. I am still a mom, with my focus on my kids and the house, I am still me, but I am much closer to being the woman that God intended me to be, so each day I rise with new hope in my heart, knowing that while I will never be perfect, every day, I am able to "strive" for that goal.

Letting go of the negativity was the first step, and as you know, a very difficult one for me. Perfectly content to complain about my life, my age, my boredom, my weight, you continued to resist the negativity I brought into your gym. You were persistent and patient with me, Armando. Constantly but gently reminding me that there was always another way to look at any situation. At first this frustrated me more than inspired me, but ultimately, I trusted you and started to believe that what you said was true. That there was something so much more for me on the other side of the walls I had built to protect myself from pain and discomfort.

I learned through you to acknowledge my behaviors and get to the root of them, and in doing so I discovered my biggest obstacle was loneliness. I would use anything from food to alcohol to people to mask that truth until I understood the difference between my truth and the Truth, which was that I am not alone at all. God has been with me all along, guiding me, leading me back to Him.

Now I no longer seek my purpose, but I do live with purpose. I live with intention. It's not about what we do, what our job title is or how much money we make. These things outside ourselves that I used to believe defined who I was; it's about, who I am to God. I have searched my entire life to discover my true purpose, what I was supposed to do with my life, completely missing the point. It's not about what to do, but who to be.

I have seen changes in you as well. Especially after that day in Litchfield when it was revealed to you that all this time, that guiding voice in your head was God. His gift to you for paying attention to that voice, for acknowledging all the things He sent you. You never dismissed anything as coincidence. And you taught me to open my eyes to the wonders of the world, the little ways God speaks to us, through a butterfly or a hummingbird, a kind word from a friend. Nothing goes unnoticed or unappreciated by you, and you have been richly rewarded, blessed, in fact.

Change is never easy. I used to think I could find the quick fix, the easy way out, but it wasn't until I faced my fears head on, and pushed through them that I was able to transform. My relationship with food and alcohol is forever different. Never again will I use these substances to hide from my pain. By being consciously aware of my feelings, I have come to a place of unconscious awareness. Maintaining my weight is no longer something I think about. I have been freed Armando. Freed to move forward. And while I still have challenges to face, demons to overcome, I no longer dread the challenges; I welcome them for I know there is something good beyond them. A peace beyond all understanding and that is something worth fighting for.

Sincerely,
Debbie Bohling

"Therefore, everyone who hears these words of mine and puts them into practice is like a wise man who built his house on the rock. The rain came down, the streams rose, and the winds blew and beat against the house; yet it did not fall, because it had its **solid foundation** *on the rock. But everyone who hears these words of mine and does not put them into practice is like a foolish man who built his house on sand. The rain came down, the streams rose, and the winds blew and beat against that house, and it fell with a great crash."*
Matthew 7:24-27 NIV

Your foundation has been built. Enjoy the journey! ☺

"Because you know that the testing of your faith develops perseverance. Perseverance must finish its work so that you may be mature and complete, not lacking anything. If any of you lack wisdom, he should ask God, who gives generously to all without finding fault, and it will be given to him. But when he asks, he must believe and not doubt, because he who doubts is like a wave of the sea, blown and tossed to the wind."

James 1:3-6 NIV

Conclusion

We tend to look elsewhere for answers, chasing our own tails, driving ourselves crazy when the answer is often right in front of us. Many of us focus on everything else in life other than what is most important. Slow down. Be still and listen. Listen to what is within. Look in the mirror and search. Look deep within and ask for God's grace to unleash the strength and purity he has instilled in you. He will answer, and you will find that your happiness isn't solely about losing weight. God reveals himself in the most mysterious ways. Our faith grows differently and immeasurably. Our bodies will shed pounds none the same. Our lives take different turns but will always lead us to where we are supposed to be when we seek the truth. Don't ever give up. Have faith and keep moving forward. Life is a journey and we are in control of which direction we choose to take. God will guide you and God will reveal the answers to you. Weight loss is secondary to what you will discover. Life is about living every day with joy. Share His grace, His love, and the Word with your family and friends, with a complete stranger or neighbor. Seek to find your purpose and live your passions. Share them with the world.

Life is not about denying a piece of cake at your own child's birthday party or about finding happiness and comfort in foods that are not conducive to your health and well being. It's about acknowledging, becoming aware of all that's around you, and doing things in moderation. We can live a full, balanced, vibrant life. The approach that you will take is timeless and will be effortless in time. All it takes is one moment to hear and acknowledge the truth. It is up to you if you chose to listen and then seek to live the truth to reach your divine destiny. *BELIEVE!* You will continue to grow every day for the rest of your life. Remember, it is not about being perfect; it is about striving for perfection.

Every single person is blessed with love in their hearts and the ability to live a fulfilling peaceful existence. Your new life, your full life, is waiting for you. Trust in God to guide you and you will find that taking care of your body physically and eating healthy foods from the earth will come naturally. You will know the way but know that you are not going at it alone. Now is the time to share your gifts. Share your goodness. Share your love for each other. Embrace your love for yourself. God wants you to **live the life you were meant to live.**

May God bless each and every single one of you and your families who seek the truth, hear the truth, and act on the truth: *"the truth shall set you free." John 8:32 NIV* It is your grace and faith within that brings beauty to our world.

Love,

Armando Aversa

P.S. Be persistently patient and patiently persistent. Live the truth. Your rewards and your miracles will be revealed.

"I tell you the truth, if anyone says to this mountain, 'Go throw yourself into the sea,' and does not doubt in his heart but believes that what he says will happen, it will be done for him. Therefore, I tell you, whatever you ask for in prayer, believe that you have received it, and it will be yours."
9 Mark 11:23-24 NIV

"May God's grace and peace be with you."
1 Corinthians 1:3 NIV

*"Blessed are those who have not seen
and yet have believed."*

The truth will prevail.

ACKNOWLEDGEMENTS

First and foremost, I would like to thank God for guiding me throughout my life and giving me the opportunity and the strength to persevere with delivering this message.

To my beautiful mother who is one of the most caring, up lifting, and spiritual people I have ever met. You have been an inspiration to me. Because of you, I have found true happiness. You made me *Believe* in achieving whatever my dreams and goals are in life. It is because of you I was able to seek out my true passion.

To my father, a truly amazing person, knowledgeable in all facets of life, always seeking perfection, always right even when wrong. You are dedicated to perfection; you are not obsessive, but you are eager to learn and accumulate knowledge. Thank you for guiding me and instilling in me all of your great qualities, your work ethic, dedication, passion, persistence, and desire. You are an amazing person.

To my brother Joe, the plumber, you will always be my best friend, my heart and soul. Remember that we have not grown distant; all we have done is grown up. Your work ethic is astounding, and you show nothing but pure joy in each of your accomplishments. If our world had your work ethic, it would be a better place. The sky is the limit. Thank you for being the best brother a guy could ever have.

To my sister, Patricia. Oh, dear sister, where are you? I hope this message finds you well as I remember you only from my younger days. I am confident you will overcome the situations you are in, and I know you will fight through the temptations that you have fallen into. I dedicated a direct message to you in this book and hope it finds you. Thank you for being the sister you were, and I am looking forward to seeing you become the sister you always wanted to be. I Believe in my heart that if this message finds you, you will then find the missing link to your success.

Antonella, if you only knew how much you have opened my eyes and how much I learned from having a relationship with you. I've wanted to be so much like you when I was going in the wrong direction in life. You showed me the value of being wholesome. You were nurturing, caring, giving, and sweet--qualities I had possessed but that were dormant. You opened my eyes to how one should be. You deserve the world, and I am forever grateful for you coming into my life. You will always hold a special place in my heart. I will always be here for you for whatever it is that you need in life.

One of my closest friends, Tom Murtha. You may not know the magnitude and impact that you have made on my life, but I am here to say that without you all of this could not have been possible. You were the foundation. It was you who made me *Believe* in myself. Thank you for guiding me and helping me learn how to build my own home, and thank you for instilling in me the knowledge of how to grow as a person.

To Jon Doyle, the qualities you possess in a friend and in a person have truly been inspirational. The knowledge you possess in the health field is astounding. I have seen you accomplish what you set out to do and what you are most passionate about. You never stopped, and to see the persistence you portrayed and the dedication you have shown toward growth as a human is truly remarkable. You set goals in your life, and you reach them. You inspired me by modeling success. You always guided me and put me on the right track. You played a huge factor in this book, and I can't thank you enough for all that you have done throughout the years.

Debbie, what you have accomplished from the day I met you was remarkable and empowering, although your transformation was natural and simple. I cannot express my thanks adequately for your support, your belief in me, and for the letter that I received from you. Your letter inspired me to reach the tens of millions who are in a similar place as you were when we met.

I cannot express my gratitude for having the pleasure to know the Bohling Family. I want to thank you for all of the support each of you have shown me throughout this journey. It has been greatly appreciated, and I value the friendship we have established.

To Michelle Marella, no acknowledgment is powerful enough to express how fortunate I feel to have you as a friend and business partner in delivering this book!!! Thank you for all that you do!!! You are a Godsend!!!

To Michael Strozier and Kyle Torke of World Audience Publishers, without the both of you my words would not have been shared with the world. It is because of your guidance that I have been able to create this book in my own words. You are both very talented and gifted with what you do! Thank you for believing in me and my story and allowing me to express this message to the world.

To one of my closest friends from college, Ryan Goldsby. You always believed in me and lifted me at times I needed support. You *Believe* in following your heart and being a good person, and you are one who has incredible qualities instilled in yourself that every individual should possess. Although you live so far away, you will always be so close in my heart.

I would like to give special thanks to my clients, to all of you for all that you have done, and you all know who you are. I have learned much from each and every one of you over these past ten years. It is because of you and the impact you had on my life that I have become who I am today. I paid attention to every single detail when speaking to you, and I can't thank you enough for sharing your life occurrences with me. All of you know who you are, and to address each and every one of you, the book would never end. In some way, somehow, in some sort of fashion, each of you has helped me, *Believe*.

"And Jesus grew in wisdom and stature, and in favor with God and man."
Luke 2:52 NIV

To you fathers and men in this world, this message is for you as well for all that you do for your families, for all that you achieve in life, the assessments you make to make better family decisions within your homes, and your contributions to this world. You are a major part to this puzzle.

Last but not least, to all of you amazing mothers: you are the reason I have accomplished and written this book. What I've learned from all of you is priceless. Whether it be the conversations we had regarding sports bras, perms, your manicure, your straight hair, your bad haircut, your child's first tooth, your battle with cancer, or your pregnancy, every single one of our conversations was meaningful, and I gained more wisdom from you women than you could imagine.

"There is neither Jew nor Gentile, there is neither slave nor free, nor is there male or female:
for you are all one in Christ Jesus."
Gal 3:28 NIV

Before I send you off, I would like to share with you a letter I had received on February 7, 2011.

To: Armando

Here is something that crossed my mind if you ever were curious to how I think today about my life:

"GOD will restore me to sanity if I relate myself to Him"

Although we fall short, Jesus is the example we should all live by. Whenever you do something or are having trouble making choices, ask yourself, "What would Jesus do?"

My last crack episode landed me in the hospital Thanksgiving Day 2010, totally broken. It was then that I was able to see my past float in front of me. I realized that, through using crack, I had lived every nightmare I had ever had. My own self-will and obsession to smoke crack drove me into a dark pit of despair. Finally beaten, I asked for God's help. His presence told me to *Believe!* My obsession for crack has been taken away, and my paranoia has been since lifted. I am no longer afraid. I know my life is healthy and sane.

Sincerely,

Your sister who believes there is a God. Call on Him, and He will be there.

Patricia Aversa

My sister is back! ☺!!!

Now that is the power of **BELIEVE**...

Authors Note

    The wisdom I gained from training my clients, through their struggles and triumphs, is priceless. I am fortunate to have had the opportunity, and I have deep gratitude for all that I have learned from others.
    I believe the keys to your success in weight loss and achieving ultimate happiness are not only learned through your own personal experiences, but also from others—from the sharing of our tales. Along my journey I recorded many moments, thoughts, ideas, and inspirations. Some experiences I did not include but I still hold dear in my heart. As my gift to you, I would like to share the remainder of the collaboration of knowledge and wisdom I gained throughout the years at armandoarversa.com. Look for *Believe: The Holy Grail of Weight Loss* on Facebook to see a picture of a true "Holy Cow" moment! ☺ I discovered the picture just prior to the final edit of *Believe*. Gods signs never stop coming. This page was created for you to post your inspirational stories, experiences and photos after reading Believe. It's important to learn from one another!
    I hope you will attempt to stay conscious and aware of the signs and guidance you will receive when you open up your heart. I would not have been able to write this book had I not been open and unafraid to ask for God's guidance. If I were not receptive during my adventures in Newport and the Bahamas, to my thoughts while awake at 3am, and during training sessions with clients, I would have missed all of the incredible blessings and opportunity of you having read *Believe*.
    Enjoy the miracles and blessings God brings to your life. Enjoy **your** journey! My arms and my heart are open to each and every one of you. I would love to hear your feedback. Please share your story, your success, and your miracles with me!

God Bless you and your families,

Armando

Armando@armandoarversa.com

"Grace and peace be yours in abundance through the knowledge of God and of Jesus our Lord.
His divine power has given us everything we need for a godly life through our knowledge of him who called us by his own glory and goodness. Through these he has given us his very great and precious promises, so that through them you may participate in the divine nature, having escaped the corruption in the world caused by evil desires.
For this very reason, make every effort to add to your faith goodness; and to goodness, knowledge; and to knowledge, self-control; and to self-control, perseverance; and to perseverance, godliness; and to godliness, mutual affection; and to mutual affection, love. For if you possess these qualities in increasing measure, they will keep you from being ineffective and unproductive in your knowledge of our Lord Jesus Christ. But whoever does not have them is nearsighted and blind, forgetting that they have been cleansed from their past sins.
Therefore, my brothers and sisters, make every effort to confirm your calling and election. For if you do these things, you will never stumble, and you will receive a rich welcome into the eternal kingdom of our Lord and Savior Jesus Christ."
2 Peter 1 NIV

Here are a few more verses that I came across while on the journey that were meant to be shared with you.

"God is spirit, and his worshipers must worship in the Spirit and in truth."
John 4:24 NIV

"The one who gets wisdom loves life;
the one who cherishes understanding will soon prosper."
Proverbs 19:8 NIV

"But we ought always to thank God for you, brothers and sisters loved by the Lord, because God chose you as first fruits to be saved through the sanctifying work of the Spirit and through belief in the truth."
2 Thessalonians 2:13 NIV

"Finally, brothers and sisters, whatever is true, whatever is noble, whatever is right, whatever is pure, whatever is lovely, whatever is admirable—if anything is excellent or praiseworthy—think about such things. ^{9} Whatever you have learned or received or heard from me, or seen in me—put it into practice. And the God of peace will be with you." Philippians 4:8-9 NIV

*"Buy the truth and do not sell it—
wisdom, instruction and insight as well.
The father of a righteous child has great joy;
a man who fathers a wise son rejoices in him.
May your father and mother rejoice;
may she who gave you birth be joyful!"
Proverbs 23:23-25 NIV*

*"Wisdom is a shelter
as money is a shelter,
but the advantage of knowledge is this:
Wisdom preserves those who have it."
Ecclesiastes 7:12 NIV*

*"Do not merely listen to the word, and so deceive yourselves. Do what it says. Anyone who listens to the word but does not do what it says is like someone who looks at his face in a mirror and, after looking at himself, goes away and immediately forgets what he looks like. But whoever looks intently into the perfect law that gives freedom, and continues in it—not forgetting what they have heard, but doing it—they will be blessed in what they do."
James 1:22-25*

*"Very truly I tell you, whoever believes in me will do the works I have been doing, and they will do even greater things than these, because I am going to the Father."
John 14:12*

*"In everything I did, I showed you that by this kind of hard work we must help the weak, remembering the words the Lord Jesus himself said: 'It is more blessed to give than to receive."
Acts 20:35 NIV*

"Give, and it will be given to you. A good measure, pressed down, shaken together and running over, will be poured into your lap. For with the measure you use, it will be measured to you."
Luke 6:38

*"Trust in the LORD with all your heart
and lean not on your own understanding;
in all your ways submit to him,
and he will make your paths straight."*
Proverbs 3:5-6

"And we also thank God continually because, when you received the word of God, which you heard from us, you accepted it not as a human word, but as it actually is, the word of God, which is indeed at work in you who believe." 1 Thessalonians 2:13 NIV

"I am the true vine, and my Father is the gardener. He cuts off every branch in me that bears no fruit, while every branch that does bear fruit he prunes so that it will be even more fruitful. You are already clean because of the word I have spoken to you. Remain in me, as I also remain in you. No branch can bear fruit by itself; it must remain in the vine. Neither can you bear fruit unless you remain in me.
"I am the vine; you are the branches. If you remain in me and I in you, you will bear much fruit; apart from me you can do nothing. If you do not remain in me, you are like a branch that is thrown away and withers; such branches are picked up, thrown into the fire and burned. If you remain in me and my words remain in you, ask whatever you wish, and it will be done for you. This is to my Father's glory, that you bear much fruit, showing yourselves to be my disciples."
John 15:1-8 NIV

*"For you created my inmost being;
you knit me together in my mother's womb.
I praise you because I am fearfully and wonderfully made;
your works are wonderful,
I know that full well.
My frame was not hidden from you
when I was made in the secret place,*

when I was woven together in the depths of the earth.
Your eyes saw my unformed body;
all the days ordained for me were written in your book
before one of them came to be."
Psalm 139:13-16 NIV

We have different gifts, according to the grace given us. If a man's gift is prophesying, let him use it in proportion to his faith. If it is serving, let him serve; if it is teaching, let him teach; if it is encouraging, let him encourage; if it is contributing to the needs of others, let him give generously; if it is leadership, let him govern diligently; if it is showing mercy, let him do it cheerfully.
Romans 12:6-8 NIV

"Be careful not to practice your righteousness in front of others to be seen by them. If you do, you will have no reward from your Father in heaven. So when you give to the needy, do not announce it with trumpets, as the hypocrites do in the synagogues and on the streets, to be honored by others. Truly I tell you, they have received their reward in full."
Matthew 6:1-2 NIV

Jesus sat down opposite the place where the offerings were put and watched the crowd putting their money into the temple treasury. Many rich people threw in large amounts. But a poor widow came and put in two very small copper coins, worth only a few cents.
Calling his disciples to him, Jesus said, "Truly I tell you, this poor widow has put more into the treasury than all the others.
Mark 12:41-43 NIV

"The generous will themselves be blessed,
for they share their food with the poor."
Proverbs 22:9 NIV

"When you reap the harvest of your land, do not reap to the very edges of your field or gather the gleanings of your harvest. ¹⁰ Do not go over your vineyard a second time or pick up the grapes that have fallen. Leave them for the poor and the foreigner. I am the LORD your God."
Leviticus 19:9-10 NIV

*"and if you spend yourselves in behalf of the hungry
and satisfy the needs of the oppressed,
then your light will rise in the darkness,
and your night will become like the noonday.
The LORD will guide you always;
he will satisfy your needs in a sun-scorched land
and will strengthen your frame.
You will be like a well-watered garden,
like a spring whose waters never fail."
Isaiah 58:10-11 NIV*

*"Do to others as you would have them do to you.
"If you love those who love you, what credit is that to you? Even sinners love those who love them. And if you do good to those who are good to you, what credit is that to you? Even sinners do that. And if you lend to those from whom you expect repayment, what credit is that to you? Even sinners lend to sinners, expecting to be repaid in full. But love your enemies, do good to them, and lend to them without expecting to get anything back. Then your reward will be great, and you will be children of the Most High, because he is kind to the ungrateful and wicked."
Luke 6:31-35 NIV*

*"Since you died with Christ to the elemental spiritual forces of this world, why, as though you still belonged to the world, do you submit to its rules: [21] "Do not handle! Do not taste! Do not touch!"? [22] These rules, which have to do with things that are all destined to perish with use, are based on merely human commands and teachings. [23] Such regulations indeed have an appearance of wisdom, with their self-imposed worship, their false humility and their harsh treatment of the body, but they lack any value in restraining sensual indulgence."
Colossians 2:20-23 NIV*

"Please test your servants for ten days: Give us nothing but vegetables to eat and water to drink. Then compare our appearance with that of the young men who eat the royal food, and treat your servants in accordance with what you see." So he agreed to this and tested them for ten days.

At the end of the ten days they looked healthier and better nourished than any of the young men who ate the royal food. So the guard took away their choice food and the wine they were to drink and gave them vegetables instead.
To these four young men God gave knowledge and understanding of all kinds of literature and learning. And Daniel could understand visions and dreams of all kinds."
Daniel 1:12-17 NIV

"Accept the one whose faith is weak, without quarreling over disputable matters. One person's faith allows them to eat anything, but another, whose faith is weak, eats only vegetables.
The one who eats everything must not treat with contempt the one who does not, and the one who does not eat everything must not judge the one who does, for God has accepted them. Who are you to judge someone else's servant? To their own master, servants stand or fall. And they will stand, for the Lord is able to make them stand."
Romans 1-4 NIV

"My dear brothers and sisters, take note of this: Everyone should be quick to listen, slow to speak and slow to become angry, because human anger does not produce the righteousness that God desires." James 1:19-20 NIV

"Truthful lips endure forever, but a lying tongue lasts only a moment."
Proverbs 13:19 NIV

"A gentle answer turns away wrath,
but a harsh word stirs up anger."
Proverbs 15:1 NIV

"Watch out for false prophets. They come to you in sheep's clothing, but inwardly they are ferocious wolves. By their fruit you will recognize them. Do people pick grapes from thorn bushes, or figs from thistles? Likewise, every good tree bears good fruit, but a bad tree bears bad fruit. A good tree cannot bear bad fruit, and a bad tree cannot bear good fruit. Every tree that does not bear good fruit is cut down and thrown into the fire. Thus, by their fruit you will recognize them.
Matthew 7:15-20 NIV

*A fool gives full vent to his anger,
but a wise man keeps himself under control."
Proverbs 29:11 NIV*

*"Therefore, as God's chosen people, holy and dearly loved, clothe yourselves with compassion, kindness, humility, gentleness and patience. Bear with each other and forgive one another if any of you has a grievance against someone. Forgive as the Lord forgave you. And over all these virtues put on love, which binds them all together in perfect unity."
Colossians 3:12-14 NIV*

*"and all the ways that wickedness deceives those who are perishing. They perish because they refused to love the truth and so be saved."
2 Thessalonians 2:10 NIV*

*One of the teachers of the law came and heard them debating. Noticing that Jesus had given them a good answer, he asked him, "Of all the commandments, which is the most important?"
"The most important one," answered Jesus, "is this: 'Hear, O Israel: The Lord our God, the Lord is one. Love the Lord your God with all your heart and with all your soul and with all your mind and with all your strength.' The second is this: 'Love your neighbor as yourself.' There is no commandment greater than these."
Mark 12:28-31 NIV*

*"I urge you, brothers and sisters, to watch out for those who cause divisions and put obstacles in your way that are contrary to the teaching you have learned. Keep away from them. For such people are not serving our Lord Christ, but their own appetites. By smooth talk and flattery they deceive the minds of naive people. Everyone has heard about your obedience, so I rejoice because of you; but I want you to be wise about what is good, and innocent about what is evil. The God of peace will soon crush Satan under your feet.
The grace of our Lord Jesus be with you."
Romans 16:17-20 NIV*

"Be careful, however, that the exercise of your rights does not become a stumbling block to the weak. For if someone with a weak conscience sees you, with all your knowledge, eating in an idol's temple, won't that person be emboldened to eat what is sacrificed to idols? So this weak brother or sister, for whom Christ died, is destroyed by your knowledge. When you sin against them in this way and wound their weak conscience, you sin against Christ. Therefore, if what I eat causes my brother or sister to fall into sin, I will never eat meat again, so that I will not cause them to fall."
1 Corinthians 8:9-13 NIV

"Those who want to get rich fall into temptation and a trap and into many foolish and harmful desires that plunge people into ruin and destruction. ^{10} For the love of money is a root of all kinds of evil. Some people, eager for money, have wandered from the faith and pierced themselves with many griefs."
1 Timothy 6:9-11 NIV

*"Avoid it, do not travel on it;
turn from it and go on your way."*
Proverbs 4:15 NIV

"If your brother or sister is distressed because of what you eat, you are no longer acting in love. Do not by your eating destroy someone for whom Christ died."
Romans 14:15 NIV

*"He makes grass grow for the cattle,
and plants for people to cultivate—
bringing forth food from the earth."*
Psalm 104:14 NIV

"Then God said, "I give you every seed-bearing plant on the face of the whole earth and every tree that has fruit with seed in it. They will be yours for food."
Genesis 1:29 NIV

"He will be eating curds and honey when he knows enough to reject the wrong and choose the right."
Isaiah 7:15 NIV

"Stop drinking only water, and use a little wine because of your stomach and your frequent illnesses.
1 Timothy 5:23 NIV

"They are like a man building a house, who dug down deep and laid the foundation on rock. When a flood came, the torrent struck that house but could not shake it, because it was well built."
Luke 6:48 NIV

"For we are God's masterpiece. He has created a new in Christ Jesus, so we can do the good things he planned for us long ago."
Colossians 4:2 NIV

PHOTOS

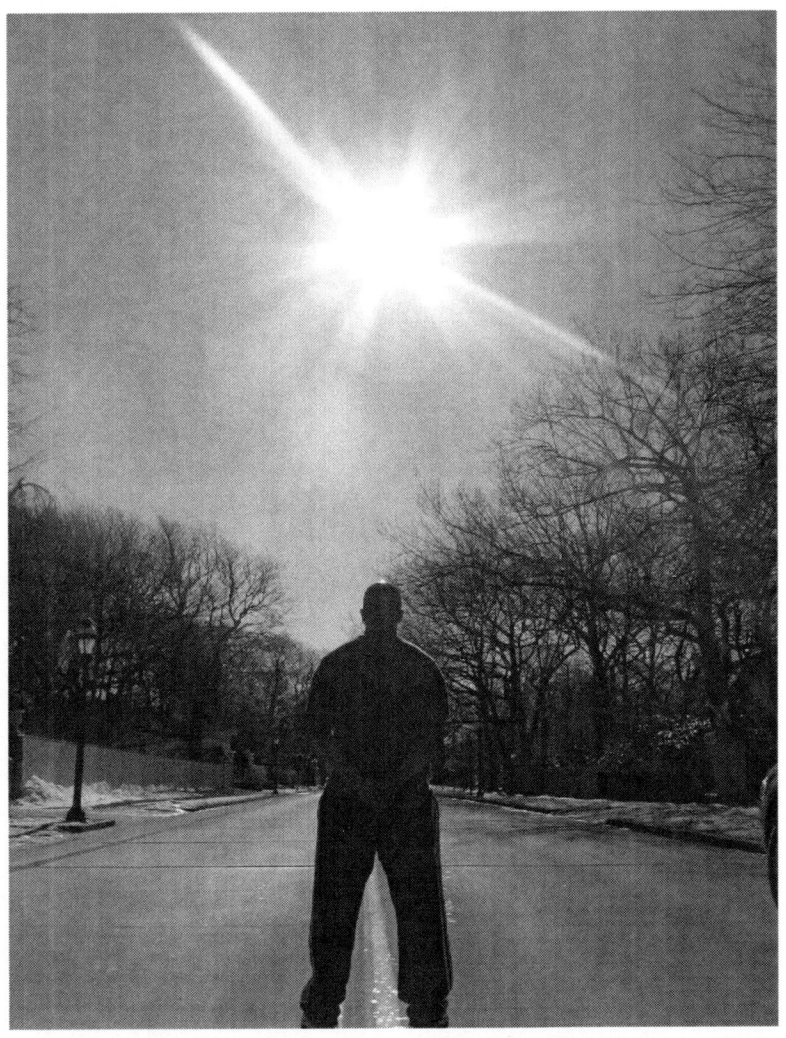

Newport, RI, on the way to The Cliff Walk.

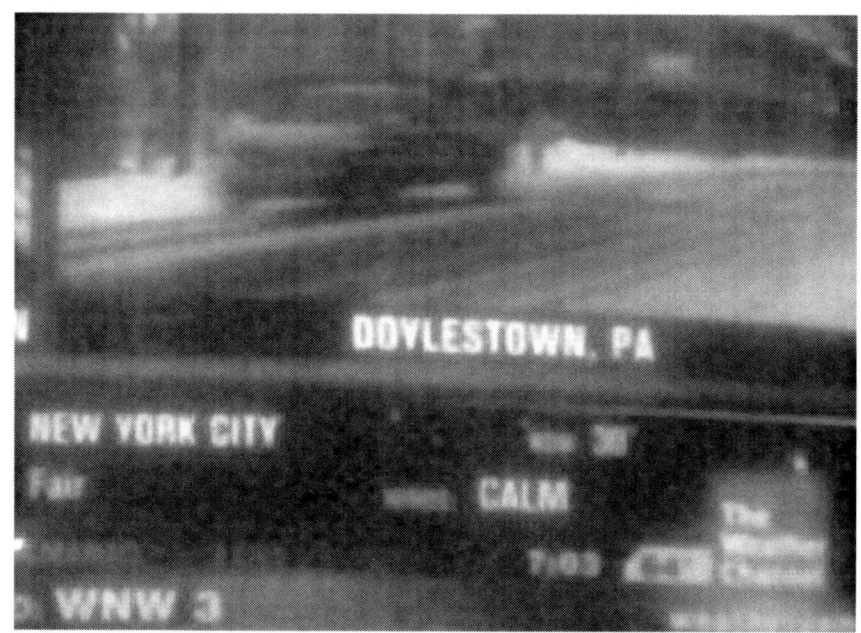

Doylestown, PA (photo taken in the Bahamas).

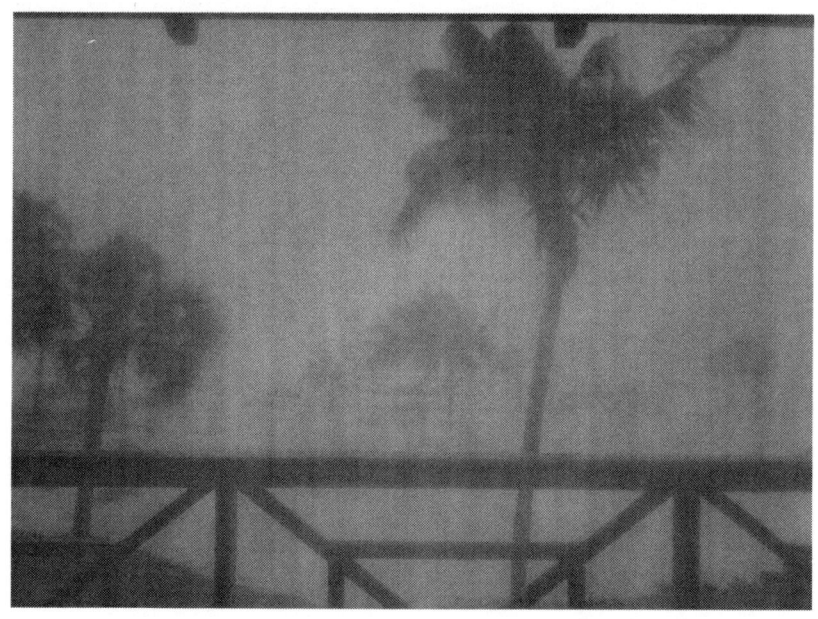

Beautiful 30° and 30 mph winds in the Bahamas.

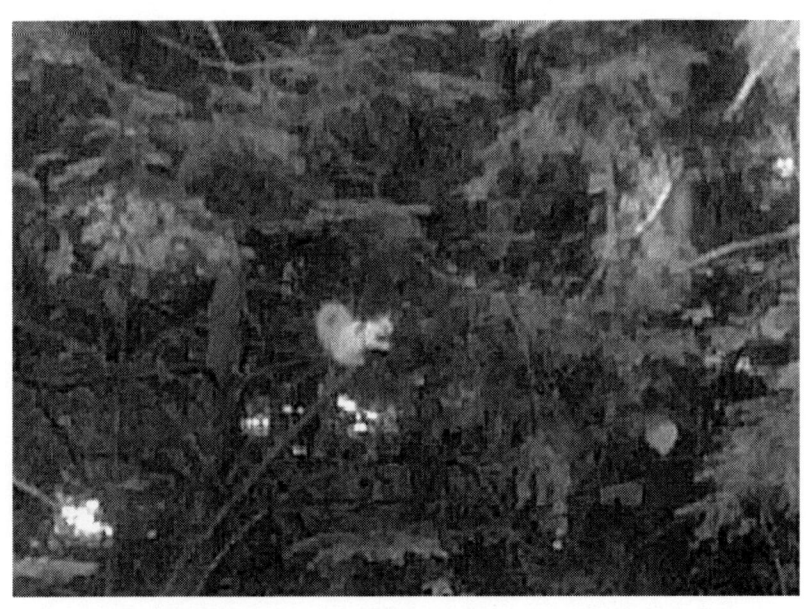

A white squirrel on my property.

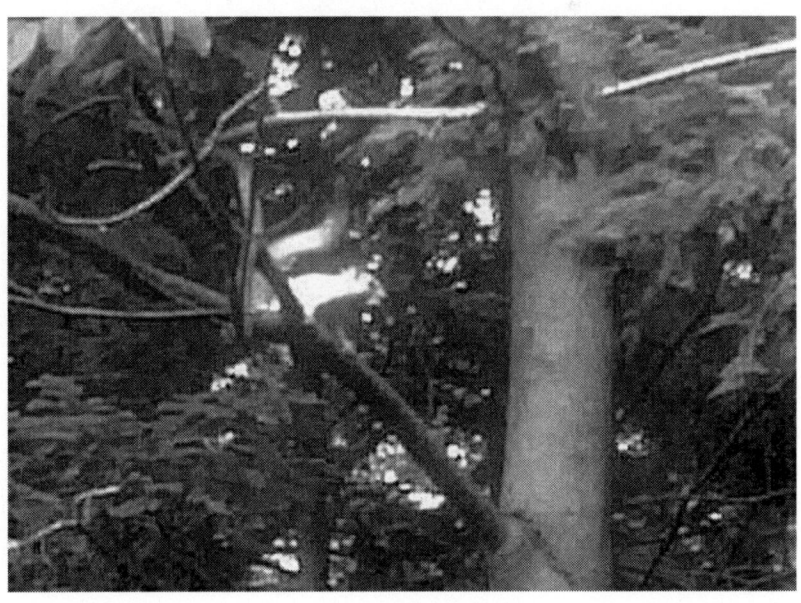

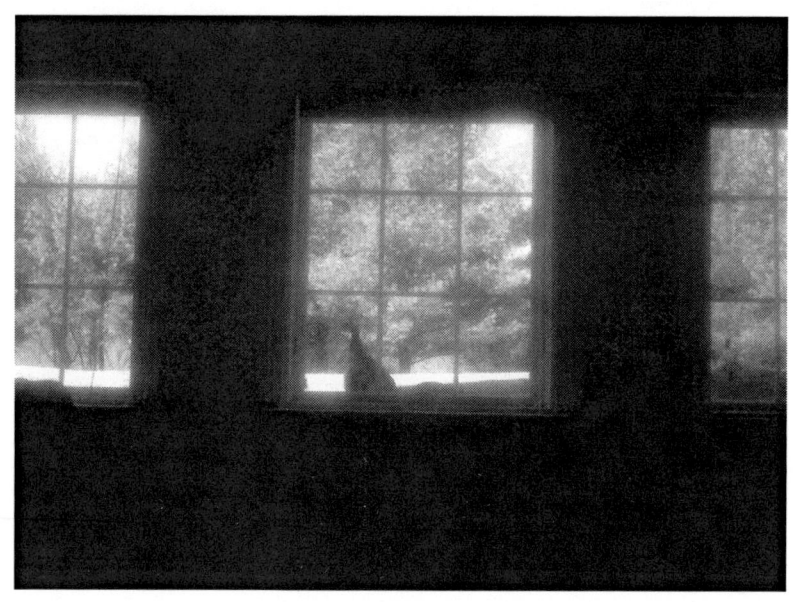

Guinea Hens on my property.

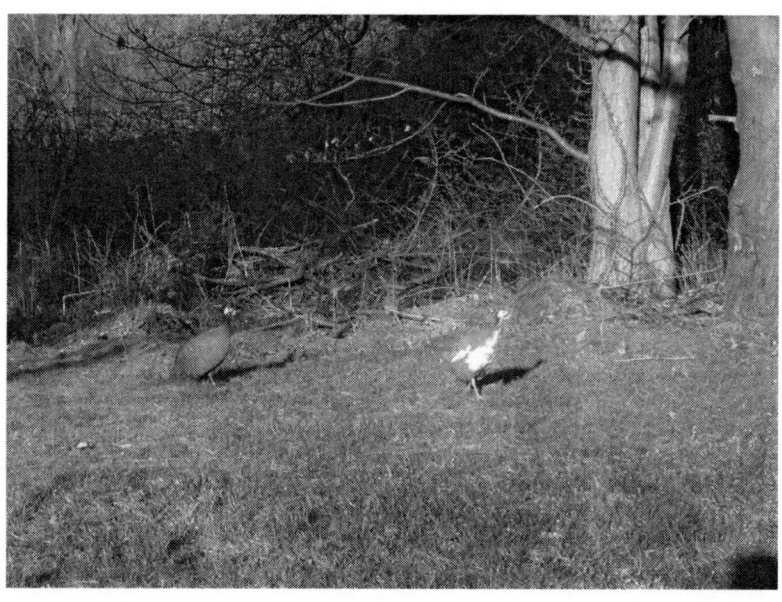

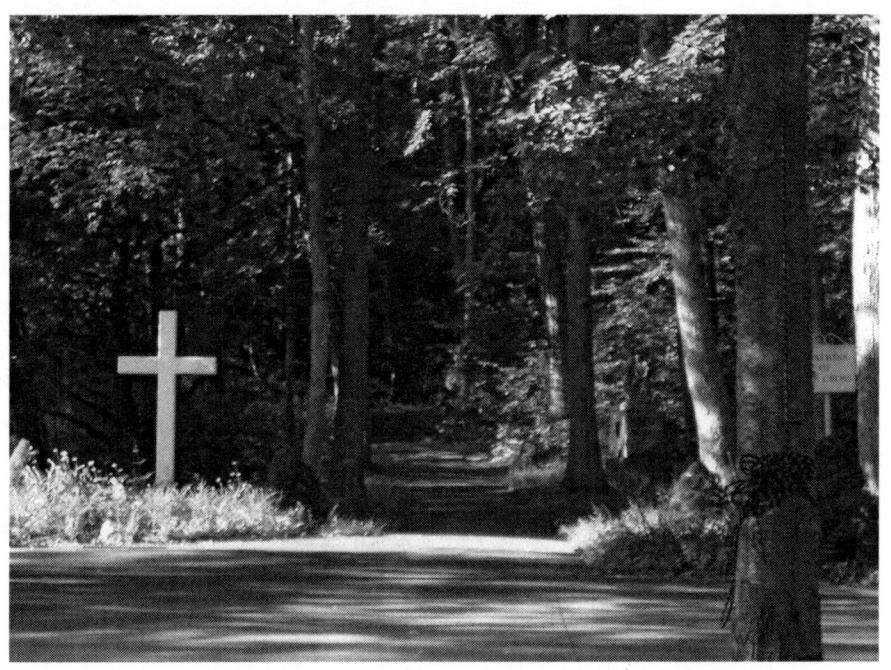

Entrance to the Stations of the Cross —"Imagine how I felt."

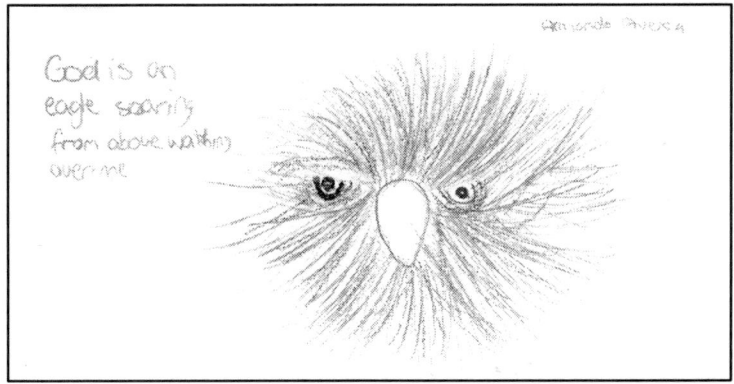

While in Newport, I found this photo in the Bible that my father had given me. I drew this when I was a child. Obviously, being an artist was not my talent.

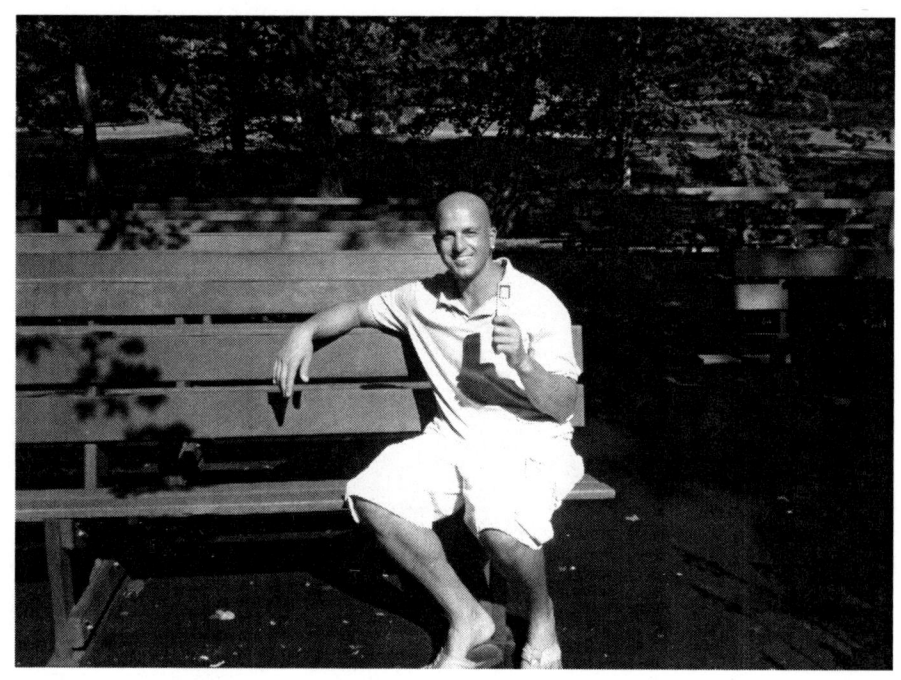

Thank God for tape recorders.

CPSIA information can be obtained at www.ICGtesting.com
262218BV00001B/6/P